Cytotoxicity - A Crucial Toxicity Test for *In Vitro* Experiments

Edited by Pinar Erkekoğlu

Published in London, United Kingdom

Cytotoxicity - A Crucial Toxicity Test for *In Vitro* Experiments
http://dx.doi.org/10.5772/intechopen.1002154
Edited by Pinar Erkekoğlu

Contributors
Alimukhamedova Orzigul Bakhrievna, Azimova Shakhnoz Sadikovna, Hare Ram Singh, Kannaiah Surendirakumar, Khamidova Umida Bakhriddin Kizi, Khashimova Zaynat Sattarovna, Manoharan Ravi, Maria Katsikogianni, Mashilo Matotoka, Mitali Singhal, Peter Masoko, Pinar Erkekoğlu, Pitchai Palaniappan, Pragya Prakash, Ramar Ramesh, Sabita Shaha, Shoaib Haidar, Terenteva Ekaterina Olegovna, Tosheva Nigora Arziyevna, Umarova Mukaddas Rustamovna, Yüksel Çetin

First published in London, United Kingdom, 2025 by IntechOpen
IntechOpen is the global imprint of INTECHOPEN LIMITED, registered in England and Wales, registration number: 11086078, 167-169 Great Portland Street, London, W1W 5PF, United Kingdom

For EU product safety concerns: IN TECH d.o.o., Prolaz Marije Krucifikse Kozulić 3, 51000 Rijeka, Croatia, info@intechopen.com or visit our website at intechopen.com.

British Library Cataloguing-in-Publication Data
A catalogue record for this book is available from the British Library

Cytotoxicity - A Crucial Toxicity Test for *In Vitro* Experiments
Edited by Pinar Erkekoğlu
p. cm.

This title is part of the Biochemistry Book Series, Volume 63
Topic: Cell and Molecular Biology
Series Editor: Andrei Surguchov
Topic Editor: Mary C. Maj
Associate Topic Editor: Felicia Ikolo

Print ISBN 978-1-83634-032-4
Online ISBN 978-1-83634-031-7
eBook (PDF) ISBN 978-1-83634-033-1
ISSN 2632-0983

IntechOpen Book Series
Biochemistry
Volume 63

Aims and Scope of the Series

Biochemistry, the study of chemical transformations occurring within living organisms, impacts all of the life sciences, from molecular crystallography and genetics, to ecology, medicine and population biology. Biochemistry studies macromolecules - proteins, nucleic acids, carbohydrates and lipids –their building blocks, structures, functions and interactions. Much of biochemistry is devoted to enzymes, proteins that catalyze chemical reactions, enzyme structures, mechanisms of action and their roles within cells. Biochemistry also studies small signaling molecules, coenzymes, inhibitors, vitamins and hormones, which play roles in the life process. Biochemical experimentation, besides coopting the methods of classical chemistry, e.g., chromatography, adopted new techniques, e.g., X-ray diffraction, electron microscopy, NMR, radioisotopes, and developed sophisticated microbial genetic tools, e.g., auxotroph mutants and their revertants, fermentation, etc. More recently, biochemistry embraced the 'big data' omics systems. Initial biochemical studies have been exclusively analytic: dissecting, purifying and examining individual components of a biological system; in exemplary words of Efraim Racker, (1913 –1991) "Don't waste clean thinking on dirty enzymes." Today, however, biochemistry is becoming more agglomerative and comprehensive, setting out to integrate and describe fully a particular biological system. The 'big data' metabolomics can define the complement of small molecules, e.g., in a soil or biofilm sample; proteomics can distinguish all the proteins comprising e.g., serum; metagenomics can identify all the genes in a complex environment e.g., the bovine rumen.
This Biochemistry Series will address both the current research on biomolecules, and the emerging trends with great promise.

Meet the Series Editor

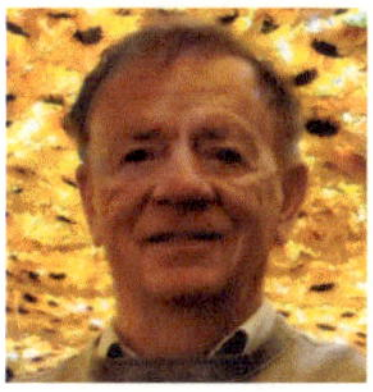

Andrei Surguchov, Ph.D., joined Baylor College of Medicine, Houston, TX, as a faculty member in 1992, where he studied the mechanisms of the genetic control of lipid metabolism. At the University of Utah, his research interests focused on cloning new genes encoding retinal proteins. He studied molecular and cellular mechanisms of neurodegenerative diseases and retinal degeneration at Washington University, St. Louis. Currently, his research focuses on the structure-function relationship of proteins involved in neurodegeneration and ocular diseases. Andrei Surguchov is an Editor-in-Chief at Biochemistry Research International and Associate Editor in several biomedical journals.

Meet the Volume Editor

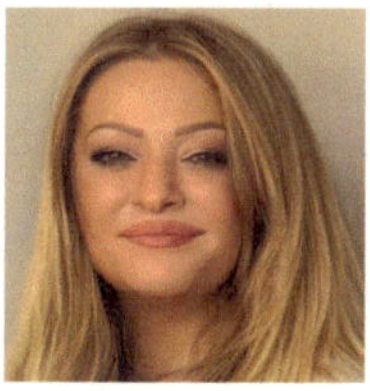

Prof. Erkekoğlu graduated from the Hacettepe University Faculty of Pharmacy in Türkiye and received her master's and Ph.D. degrees in toxicology. During her doctoral thesis, she worked at Joseph Fourier University and the Laboratory for Alloys and Nanomaterials (LAN) within the Institute for Nanoscience and Cryogenics (INAC) at the French Alternative Energies and Atomic Energy Commission (CEA) in France. She completed her postdoctoral studies at the Department of Biological Engineering at MIT. She currently serves as the Head of the Department of Pharmaceutical Toxicology at Hacettepe University. She is also a board member of Hacettepe University Vaccine Institute and Head of the Department of Vaccine Technology. In 2024, she was appointed as a scientific board member of the Türkiye Vaccine Institute. She has over 250 scientific articles published in peer-reviewed journals. She has edited ten international books and written 15 national/international book chapters.

Contents

Preface

Cytotoxicity is a term used to describe “a single toxic effect on any cell type that can cause cell death”. Some chemical, physical and biological agents may impair cellular functions and disrupt cellular membranes by directly inducing oxidative stress. Other substances may exert toxic effects through intermediary processes, such as causing an immune response that damages host cells or disrupts cellular signalling pathways. The possible harmful effects of different agents can finally lead to cell death.

Cytotoxicity is one of the first endpoints for assessing the *in vitro* toxicity of these agents, and the first test to assess their safety. Testing for cytotoxicity involves both *in vitro* and *in vivo* methods. *In vitro* methods offer a rapid and cost-effective approach using cell cultures or tissue cultures, while *in vivo* methods provide a more comprehensive assessment of living organisms.

As drugs, cosmetics and medical devices have pervasive roles in daily life and as they may lead to toxic effects and may even estranger human health, cytotoxicity tests should be performed to assess their potential toxic effects as well as their safety profiles. Rigorous cytotoxicity testing is essential for meeting regulatory standards, enhancing user safety, and improving product quality.

Ensuring the accuracy and reliability of data obtained from *in vitro* cytotoxicity studies is critical for evaluating the safety profiles of different agents. In the past years, many *in vitro* methods have been developed to evaluate the viability of cells, and each method has its advantages, disadvantages, strengths and limitations. There are different methods for determining cytotoxicity. They can be summarized as Staining Methods”, “Colorimetric Methods”, “Fluorometric Methods”, “Luminometric Methods” and “Other Methods”. “Staining Methods” are also referred to as “dye exclusion methods”, and they include Eosin, Congo Red and Erythrosine B staining. “Colorimetric Methods” include but are not limited to the MTT Test, MTS Test, XTT and WST Tests, Neutral red uptake (NRU) test, Crystal violet test, SRB Test and LDH Enzyme Release Test. The most commonly performed “Fluorometric Methods” are the alamarBlue and CFDA-AM tests. “Luminometric Methods” for determining cytotoxicity are the ATP Bioluminescence Test and Real-Time Viability Bioluminescence Test. There are also other methods, such as the MEM Elution Test, Direct Contact Method, and Agar diffusion test, for testing the cytotoxicity of different agents. The researchers should choose the most appropriate method for their research by considering the cell type they will use, the dose and properties of the chemical, physical and biological agents, and the mechanism through which it causes cell death (such as apoptosis, necrosis, autophagy).

The cytotoxicity experiments can be conducted on many types of cells with various origins, including endothelial, epithelial, or mesenchymal cells. On the other hand, the duration of the experiment, the endpoint to be measured, and the specificity and sensitivity of the method should also be considered. Further development of existing methods or development of new, easy-to-apply, rapid and accurate tests will contribute to more accurate evaluations of the cytotoxic properties of cosmetics, medical devices as well as drugs. Recent advances in alternative testing methods, such as organ-on-a-chip technologies and computational models, hold promise for bridging the gap between traditional methods and the need for more predictive and humane testing approaches. A robust cytotoxicity evaluation strategy should integrate multiple testing approaches to ensure a thorough safety assessment. By combining existing and emerging technologies, researchers and regulatory authorities can better predict and mitigate the potential risks associated with cosmetics and medical devices, thereby safeguarding public health and advancing scientific understanding.

This book mainly focuses on cytotoxicity determination as the primary and crucial step in evaluating toxicity. In this book, the readers will find traditional and new methods used to evaluate cytotoxicity. We believe that readers will get qualified scientific knowledge and a general overview of the importance of cytotoxicity testing.

I would like to thank Tea Jelaca for her enormous support and patience throughout the editorial process of this book.

Pinar Erkekoğlu
Faculty of Pharmacy,
Department of Toxicology,
Hacettepe University,
Ankara Turkey

Chapter 1

Introductory Chapter: Methods for Determining Cytotoxic Potential of Cosmetics and Medical Devices

Pinar Erkekoğlu

1. Introduction

Cosmetics and medical devices have become an integral part of our daily lives. However, rigorous assessments are required to understand the potential effects of these devices on human health and to minimize risks. In particular, determining the cytotoxicity potential of these products is of critical importance [1, 2]. Cytotoxicity testing for cosmetics and medical devices is crucial and can be conducted on various types of cells and for medical devices *in vivo* [2]. Therefore, assessing the safety of both cosmetics and medical devices is a fundamental step in determining whether the products are compatible with biological systems [3].

2. Importance of cytotoxicity in cosmetics and medical devices

Cytotoxicity refers to the ability of chemical, physical and biological agents to cause cell death, such as apoptosis, autophagy and necrosis [4]. Some agents can induce oxidative stress, leading to the generation of reactive oxygen species (ROS). Other substances may exert their toxic effects through intermediary processes, such as inducing an immune response that inadvertently damages host cells or disrupting cellular signaling pathways [5, 6].

When it comes to the assessment of the safety of cosmetics and medical devices, cytotoxicity refers to the "capability of a material being toxic to cells." Therefore, cytotoxicity experiments are conducted in order to guarantee the efficacy and safety of products. Cosmetics are applied to the skin and mucous membranes, and medical devices are usually in direct contact with body tissues. Even trace amounts of toxic substances can cause serious health problems, so comprehensive testing is essential. Many countries require cosmetic products and medical devices to undergo cytotoxicity and biocompatibility testing to meet regulatory standards. This ensures that the products are safe for consumers and guarantees that they do not cause harmful effects when used according to instructions [1, 7–10].

3. Regulations

There are various regulations and standards for safety assessments in cosmetic and medical devices worldwide. EC: 1223/2009 is the main legislation regulating the

IntechOpen

safety of cosmetic products in the European Union (EU). This regulation requires safety tests, including cytotoxicity, of cosmetic products. Before cosmetic products are put on the market, safety assessments are carried out by preparing an information file called Cosmetic Products Notification Portal (CPNP). In the USA, the Food and Drug Administration (FDA) controls the safety of cosmetic products. There is no specific guide for cytotoxicity tests in the toxicological assessment of materials used in cosmetic products. Instead, general safety tests are carried out. The ISO 10993 international standard regulation includes a series of standards for biocompatibility testing for medical devices. These standards cover the biological assessment of medical devices, including cytotoxicity tests. ISO 10993-5 gives detailed information on how to perform cytotoxicity tests *in vitro*. FDA has also accepted the necessity of compliance with International Organization for Standardization (ISO) standards in the assessment of medical devices. In the European Union, the safety and performance of medical devices are regulated by Medical Devices Regulation (MDR) EU: 2017/745. This regulation includes compliance with the ISO 10993 series, cytotoxicity and other biocompatibility tests of medical devices. Processes are subjected to various regulations and standards in different countries and regions. These regulations require comprehensive tests and evaluations to ensure the safety of products [9–15].

4. Methods for determining cytotoxicity

4.1 Staining methods

Staining methods or "dye exclusion methods" can be performed using trypan blue, Eosin, Congo red and erythrosine B [16, 17].

4.2 Colorimetric methods

The most frequently used tests among these methods are cell death/proliferation tests based on the measurement of metabolic activity (MTT (3-(4,5-dimethylthiazol-2-yl)-2,5-diphenyltetrazolium bromide), MTS (3-(4,5-dimethylthiazol-2-yl)-5-(3-carboxymethoxyphenyl)-2-(4-sulfophenyl)-2H-tetrazolium), XTT (2,3-Bis-(2-methoxy-4-nitro-5-sulfophenyl)-2H-tetrazolium carboxanilide), WST-1 (water-soluble tetrazolium 1), NRU (neutral red uptake), crystal violet, SRB (sulforhodamine B) and LDH (lactate dehydrogenase) enzyme release tests) [5].

4.3 Fluorometric methods

These tests consist of but are not limited to alamarBlue and CFDA-AM (5-carboxyfluorescein diacetate) tests [18].

4.4 Luminometric methods

Luminometric methods, which are frequently preferred in recent years, provide rapid and simple determination of cell proliferation and cytotoxicity [19]. Luminometric methods are divided into two groups: fluorescence and bioluminescence. While fluorescent substances are used in fluorescence methods, bioluminescence methods use special enzymes called luciferases and their substrates to detect live or dead cells [20]. The most commonly used luminometric methods are ATP (adenosine triphosphate) bioluminescence test and real-time viability bioluminescence test.

4.5 Other methods

The Minimal Essential Media (MEM) elution test and direct contact method and agar diffusion tests are other methods that can be used to determine cytotoxicity [19].

5. Conclusion

Determination of cytotoxicity provides the first step in obtaining *in vitro* toxicological data for the evaluation of the toxic effects' potential for cosmetics and medical devices. Cytotoxicity tests serve as a fundamental tool for evaluating the behavior of substances with potential therapeutic applications or unknown toxic effects, providing essential insights for subsequent animal or clinical trials. Consequently, ensuring the accuracy and reliability of data obtained from such studies is of critical importance. In the past years, many methods have been developed to evaluate the viability of cells and each method has its own advantages, disadvantages, strengths and limitations. In this case, the researchers should choose the most appropriate method for their research by taking into account the cell type they will use, the dose and properties of the chemical, physical and biological agents, and the mechanism through which it causes cell death (such as apoptosis, necrosis and autophagy). On the other hand, the duration of the experiment, the endpoint to be measured and the specificity and sensitivity of method should also be considered. Further development of existing methods or development of new, easy-to-apply, rapid and accurate tests will contribute to more accurate evaluations of the cytotoxic properties of cosmetics, medical devices and drugs. Recent advances in alternative testing methods, such as organ-on-a-chip technologies and computational models, hold promise for bridging the gap between traditional methods and the need for more predictive and humane testing approaches. Ultimately, a robust cytotoxicity evaluation strategy should integrate multiple testing approaches to ensure a thorough assessment of safety. By combining existing and emerging technologies, researchers and regulatory authorities can better predict and mitigate the potential risks associated with cosmetics and medical devices, thereby safeguarding public health and advancing scientific understanding.

Author details

Pinar Erkekoğlu[1,2]

1 Department of Pharmaceutical Toxicology, Ankara, Turkey

2 Department of Vaccine Technology, Hacettepe Vaccine Institute, Ankara, Turkey

*Address all correspondence to: erkekp@yahoo.com

References

[1] Räägel H, Turley A, Fish T, Franson J, Rollins T, Campbell S, et al. Medical device industry approaches for addressing sources of failing cytotoxicity scores. Biomedical Instrumentation & Technology. 2021;**55**(2):69-84. DOI: 10.2345/0899-8205-55.2.69

[2] Zhang Y. Cell toxicity mechanism and biomarker. Clinical and Translational Medicine. 2018;**7**(1):34. DOI: 10.1186/s40169-018-0212-7

[3] Gupta V, Mohapatra S, Mishra H, Farooq U, Kumar K, Ansari MJ, et al. Nanotechnology in cosmetics and cosmeceuticals—A review of latest advancements. Gels. 2022;**8**(3):173. DOI: 10.3390/gels8030173

[4] Galluzzi L, Aaronson SA, Abrams J, Alnemri ES, Andrews DW, Baehrecke EH, et al. Guidelines for the use and interpretation of assays for monitoring cell death in higher eukaryotes. Cell Death and Differentiation. 2009;**16**(8):1093-1107. DOI: 10.1038/cdd.2009.44

[5] Riss TL, Moravec RA, O'brien MA, Hawkins EM, Niles A. Homogeneous multiwell assays for measuring cell viability, cytotoxicity, and apoptosis. In: Minor LK, editor. Handbook of Assay Development in Drug Discovery. CRC Press, LLC; 2006. pp. 385-405

[6] Niles AL, Moravec RA, Eric Hesselberth P, Scurria MA, Daily WJ, Riss TL. A homogeneous assay to measure live and dead cells in the same sample by detecting different protease markers. Analytical Biochemistry. 2007;**366**(2):197-206. DOI: 10.1016/j.ab.2007.04.007

[7] Longo-Sorbello GSA, Saydam G, Banerjee D, Bertino JR. Cytotoxicity and cell growth assays. In: Celis JE, editor. Cell Biology: A Laboratory Handbook. Burlington: Elseiver Academic Press; 2006. pp. 315-325

[8] Fan F, Wood KV. Bioluminescent assays for high-throughput screening. Assay and Drug Development Technologies. 2007;**5**(1):127-136. DOI: 10.1089/adt.2006.053

[9] Liu X, Rodeheaver DP, White JC, Wright AM, Walker LM, Zhang F, et al. A comparison of in vitro cytotoxicity assays in medical device regulatory studies. Regulatory Toxicology and Pharmacology. 2018;**97**:24-32. DOI: 10.1016/j.yrtph.2018.06.003

[10] Kanďárová H, Pôbiš P. The "Big Three" in biocompatibility testing of medical devices: Implementation of alternatives to animal experimentation-are we there yet? Frontiers in Toxicology. 2024;**5**:1337468. DOI: 10.3389/ftox.2023.1337468

[11] Regulation (EC) No 1223/2009 of the European Parliament and of the Council of 30 November 2009 on Cosmetic Products [Internet]. Available from: https://health.ec.europa.eu/system/files/2016-11/cosmetic_1223_2009_regulation_en_0.pdf

[12] ISO 10993-1:2018. Biological Evaluation of Medical Devices Part 1: Evaluation and Testing within a Risk Management Process. 5th ed. Geneva: International Organization for Standardization; 2018. p. 41

[13] ISO 10993-5:2009. Biological Evaluation of Medical Devices Part 5: Tests for In Vitro Cytotoxicity. 3rd ed. Geneva: International Organization for Standardization; 2009. p. 34

[14] ISO 10993-12:2021. Biological Evaluation of Medical Devices Part 12: Sample Preparation and Reference Materials. 5th ed. Geneva: International Organization for Standardization; 2021. p. 1

[15] FDA. Recognized Consensus Standards: Medical Devices [Internet]. 2016. Available from: https://www.accessdata.fda.gov/scripts/cdrh/cfdocs/cfstandards/detail.cfm?standard__identification_no=36819

[16] Adan A, Kiraz Y, Baran Y. Cell proliferation and cytotoxicity assays. Current Pharmaceutical Biotechnology. 2016;**17**(14):1213-1221. DOI: 10.2174/1389201017666160808160513

[17] Strober W. Trypan blue exclusion test of cell viability. Current Protocols in Immunology. 2015;**111**:A3.B.1-A3.B.3. DOI: 10.1002/0471142735.ima03bs111

[18] Eilenberger C, Kratz SRA, Rothbauer M, Ehmoser EK, Ertl P, Küpcü S. Optimized alamarBlue assay protocol for drug dose-response determination of 3D tumor spheroids. MethodsX. 2018;**5**:781-787. DOI: 10.1016/j.mex.2018.07.011

[19] Aslantürk ÖS. In vitro cytotoxicity and cell viability assays: Principles, advantages, and disadvantages. In: Larramendy M, Soloneski S, editors. Genotoxicity—A Predictable Risk to Our Actual Worl. London, UK, Crotia: InTech; 2018. pp. 1-17

[20] Corey MJ, Kinders RJ, Brown LG, Vessella RL. A very sensitive coupled luminescent assay for cytotoxicity and complement-mediated lysis. Journal of Immunological Methods. 1997;**207**(1):43-51. DOI: 10.1016/s0022-1759(97)00098-7

Chapter 2

Assessing the Toxic Potential of New Entities: The Role of Cytotoxicity Assays

Yüksel Çetin

Abstract

Conducting cytotoxicity assays is crucial to assess the efficacy and safety of chemicals, pharmaceuticals, cosmetics, nanoparticles, biological agents, biomaterials, and medical devices on living cells. These assays contribute to safety profiles in various fields like pharmacology, toxicology, drug development, and environmental science by evaluating the potential risks or therapeutic benefits of different compounds. *In vitro*, cytotoxicity testing for preliminary screening of novel drugs and vaccine candidates, medical devices, bioactive compounds, waste hazard identification, the toxicity of food contaminants and residues, etc., has a vital importance in the way of its convenience, cost-effectiveness, practicality, power, and sufficiently sensitiveness enough for application in high-throughput screening and predictive means of characterizing the toxic potential of new entities. To obtain useful results that might be very critical for further investigation, selected tools for cytotoxicity testing, such as *in vitro* cell culture systems originated from the target, seeding cell density, dissolving solution for samples, tested dose ranges, exposure time and conditions, etc., have an essential role; therefore, each parameter should be applied considering natural exposure scenarios. Cytotoxicity assays can provide insights into the mechanisms of cell death or damage. Understanding these mechanisms can help predict potential side effects and guide modifications to improve safety.

Keywords: cytotoxicity, safety of chemicals, biocompatibility, nanosafety, *in vitro* testing

1. Introduction

A strategy for establishing cytotoxicity testing for chemicals with limited data relies on a recently proposed generic Adverse Outcome Pathway (AOP) from chemical exposure to cell death. Basal cytotoxicity refers to the capacity of a chemical substance to harm living cells, particularly by disrupting essential functional and structural cellular processes related to general maintenance. Chemicals can induce cell damage through various mechanisms, which may involve specific events such as the changed activation of ion channels or receptors [1]. The selection of appropriate cellular systems [2, 3] and cytotoxicity assay methods [4–6] are crucial factors in obtaining valuable results. Additionally, the implementation of testing conditions, including handling of cellular systems, cell seeding density, cultivation conditions, cell culture medium composition, selection of exposure conditions [7, 8], applied dose range, and solvent solutions for chemical agents, are critical parameters that significantly influence the outcomes.

The 7th Amendment to the EU Cosmetics Directive, which came into effect in 2013, prohibits the marketing of animal-tested cosmetics within the EU. Consequently, the demand for *in vitro* testing of cosmetic ingredients and products has significantly increased for their safety evaluation [9, 10]. Commercially available reconstructed human epidermis models have been utilized to assess the cytotoxicity, irritation, and corrosivity of cosmetic substances. These evaluations are typically conducted using 3-(4,5-dimethylthiazol-2-yl)-2,5-diphenyltetrazolium bromide (MTT) and 3T3-Neutral Red Uptake (NRU) assays, which can also be employed to determine the starting dose for acute oral toxicity testing [9–12].

Biocompatibility testing is essential for verifying the safety use of medical devices by determining their compatibility using cellular systems and identifying any potential to cause harm or adverse reactions [13]. Cytocompatibility tests specifically examine the biological response of living cells to biomaterial extracts, assessing factors such as cell viability, growth, and metabolic activity [14]. Typically, medical devices are evaluated as extracts prepared by immersing the device or its components in a suitable extraction solvent such as physiological saline, vegetable oil, or cell culture medium under controlled conditions. This extraction method is a standardized approach to assess the biocompatibility of medical devices by evaluating the release of substances that might interact with biological systems [15]. Advancing and implementing these models could greatly improve the reliability of cytotoxicity assessments, especially for devices containing low-level toxic components that are poorly soluble in polar solvents. This strategy would provide more accurate predictions of long-term safety and efficacy, better aligning *in vitro* testing with real-world device applications [16, 17].

Nanomaterials (NMs) have become increasingly used in daily life due to their extensive benefits, with applications spanning biomedicine, engineering, food, cosmetics, sensing, and energy. However, the rising production of NMs also raises the likelihood of their release into the environment, making human exposure unavoidable. The potential toxicity or environmental and human health impacts of nanoparticles (NPs) can be initially evaluated using *in vitro* cell models. Nevertheless, conventional cytotoxicity assays, such as the MTT assay, have limitations, including potential interference with the NPs being studied [18]. When designing NPs for biomedical or other applications, it is crucial to consider their physicochemical properties—such as size, shape, surface functionalization, surface chemistry, and chemical composition—since these properties can significantly influence their interactions with cell membranes and organelles at the bionano interface, which can affect cellular uptake and the resulting nanotoxicity. Additionally, another key factor contributing to NP toxicity is cytotoxicity, which depends on the quality of the nanoparticles, their sites of deposition, and the mode of administration [19].

2. Cytotoxicity testing for bioefficacy and safety of chemicals and pharmaceuticals

Evaluation of efficacy and safety is a prerequisite prior to the introduction of new chemicals in drug development. In pharmaceutical research to identify potentially harmful effects at an early stage, cytotoxicity tests are used to screen novel drug

DOI: http://dx.doi.org/10.5772/intechopen.1008309

candidates to avoid the risk of adverse reactions later in the development stage by using relevant *in vitro* models for targeting mechanisms. Therefore, it can save time and resources by eliminating potentially harmful compounds before they reach preclinical and clinical trials. Cytotoxicity tests help determine the dose-response relationship of a drug, establishing the concentration at which the drug becomes toxic to cells. This information is crucial for setting safe dosage levels for further testing and eventual clinical use. During the drug discovery process, cytotoxicity testing helps screen multiple candidate compounds, allowing researchers to focus on those with the most promising safety profiles. Cytotoxicity assays can provide insights into the mechanisms by which a drug induces cell death or damage. Understanding these mechanisms can help predict potential side effects and guide modifications to improve safety. Cytotoxicity tests can guide the optimization of drug formulations, such as the selection of excipients and delivery systems that minimize toxic effects while maximizing therapeutic efficacy. In combination with other *in vitro* and in vivo tests, cytotoxicity assays contribute to a comprehensive preclinical safety evaluation, helping to identify and mitigate risks before clinical trials. Cytotoxicity testing allows researchers to compare the safety profiles of new drugs with existing treatments. This comparative analysis can help highlight potential advantages or disadvantages of new compounds. Regulatory agencies require extensive safety data, including cytotoxicity results, before approving new drugs for clinical trials and market release.

A significant tool utilized in predictive toxicology is the adverse outcome pathway (AOP) framework, which is a conceptual model that illustrates the existing knowledge about the connection between a molecular initiating event (MIE) and an adverse outcome (AO) through a series of key events (KEs) at a biological level relevant to risk assessment. AOPs have multiple applications in non-animal chemical risk assessment, such as facilitating read-across methods, integrating approaches to testing and assessment, applying quantitative structure-activity relationships, and developing prioritization strategies [1]. To establish basal *in vitro* cytotoxicity testing for chemicals with limited data, a strategy based on a newly proposed generic AOP from chemical exposure to cell death is employed. Basal cytotoxicity refers to a chemical substance's capacity to harm living cells, particularly by disrupting functional and structural elements related to general cellular maintenance. Chemicals can induce cell damage through various mechanisms, potentially involving a specific event like the altered activation of an ion channel [20, 21] or a receptor [20, 22]. However, a general AOP from chemical exposure to cell death should ideally include more comprehensive processes that immediately disturb cellular homeostasis. One primary mechanism involves compromising plasma membrane integrity, which is largely maintained by a robust double phospholipid layer. Chemical-induced damage to this plasma membrane can occur in several ways, with accumulation and binding to the phospholipid bilayer—known as narcosis—being a prominent example [23]. Another mechanism is the disruption of subcellular structural organization, which can undermine overall cellular functionality [21, 24]. A third mechanism includes directly impairing cellular energy production, particularly by targeting mitochondria. Chemicals may disrupt the mitochondrial respiratory chain, inhibit adenosine triphosphate (ATP) synthesis, damage mitochondrial DNA, interfere with mitochondrial DNA replication, or reduce the synthesis and stability of mitochondrial transcripts [25, 26].

Set up of AOP-based *in vitro* testing of basal cytotoxicity: In case of lack of any pre-existing information on potential toxicity of a test compound toward a specific cell type. A general cytotoxicity testing scheme could be set up supported by the proposed generic AOP from chemical insult to cell death. A number of factors related to the selection of the cellular system, cytotoxicity assays, and exposure conditions must be considered prior to organizing such default *in vitro* cytotoxicity testing trials.

Selection of the cellular system: A prerequisite for reliably predicting human real-life cytotoxicity is the use of an *in vitro* system in which all critical biological targets, as depicted in the generic AOP from chemical insult to cell death, are phenotypically expressed at an in vivo-like level for the entire testing regime. Human-based *in vitro* models are obviously strongly preferred, although this may be limited because of ethical, financial, and other reasons [2, 3]. As the human body consists of a large repertoire of cell types, the selection of the cellular origin of the *in vitro* model therefore is another critical parameter.

Cell lines are more commonly utilized than primary cells for cytotoxicity testing due to their virtually limitless supply, better reproducibility, and lower labor requirements compared to many primary cell systems, which can suffer from rapid dedifferentiation [3]. Various human and rodent cell lines, including human embryonic kidney HEK293 cells, human T-cell leukemia Jurkat cells, human neuroblastoma SH-SY5Y cells, mouse neuroblastoma N2a cells, mouse embryonic NIH3T3 fibroblasts, and rat hepatoma H-4-II-E cells, have been shown sensitivity to chemical-induced cytotoxicity [27]. However, it's important to note that many cell lines are derived from cancerous tissues, which can result in abnormal functionality, particularly in the biotransformation machinery that may be crucial for the activation or deactivation of chemicals [2, 3]. Benefits of using cell lines include reduced cellular and material costs and high-throughput capabilities. Key factors in setting up cytotoxicity assays include cell seeding density [8, 28], cultivation on extracellular matrix scaffolds [29], and the composition of the cell culture medium, including supplements like serum to enhance cell attachment [30]. Since many cytotoxicity assays measure the release of cellular components into the culture medium over time, the frequency of media renewal and the timing of sampling should be carefully planned.

Selection of cytotoxicity assays: For chemicals without existing toxicological data, *in vitro* cytotoxicity testing can rely on the proposed generic AOP pathway. Mitochondria are crucial biomarkers of chemical-induced cellular damage due to their central role in the initiation and progression of cytotoxicity. A summary of commonly used cytotoxicity assays, including their mechanisms, benefits, and limitations, is provided in **Table 1** [4–6]. For chemicals without existing toxicological data, *in vitro* cytotoxicity testing can rely on the proposed generic AOP pathway. Mitochondria are crucial biomarkers of chemical-induced cellular damage due to their central role in the initiation and progression of cytotoxicity. A summary of commonly used cytotoxicity assays, including their mechanisms, benefits, and limitations, is provided in **Table 1** [4–6]. The [3-(4,5-dimethylthiazol-2-yl)-2,5-diphenyltetrazolium bromide] (MTT) assay is widely used; it is a colorimetric method that measures the reduction of a yellow tetrazolium salt to a blue insoluble formazan, which is retained in viable cells [31]. The mitochondrial enzyme succinate dehydrogenase is responsible for this reduction. The MTT assay reflects mitochondrial integrity and activity, providing an indication of cell viability and number. The amount of formazan produced is proportional to the number of surviving cells, and IC50 values are typically determined, representing the concentration of the test compound that causes cell death in 50% of the cultured cells [32].

A number of other tetrazolium salts, such as 3-(4,5-dimetiltiyazol-2-yl)-5-(3-karboksimetoksifenil)-2-(4-sülfofenil)-2H-tetrazolyum (MTS), 2,3-bis-(2-metoksi-4-nitro-5-sülfofenil)-2H-tetrazolyum-5-karboksianilid (XTT), and 2-(4-iodofenil)-3-(4-nitrofenil)-5-(2,4-disülfofenil)-2H-tetrazolyum (WST) can be

Method	Mechanism of action	Advantages	Disadvantages
XTT MTS WST MTT	Mitochondrial activity Reduction of formazan via NADH electron transfer to form MTT	Proper for potential drug follow-up studies Widely used Inexpensive Sensitive response to the cell proliferation Rapid preliminary screening WST eliminates the needs for washing and less toxic Fast, easy-to-handle, low-cost model with wide use and reproducible results	Long-time incubation Steps in protocol (MTT) Toxic to cell Not suitable for long-term studies Limited sensitivity Work with high cell numbers Cannot differ cytotoxic or cytostatic Not suitable for suspending cells Several interferences depend on the compounds used, such reducing agent
Neutral red uptake assay	Viable cells bind to the dye and attach themselves by hydrophobic electrostatic bonds to anionic sites in the lysosomal matrix	May have some interference of test compound In vitro/in vivo correlation in the 95% range; low cost, no unstable reagents	Enumeration of cells is not dependent on enzymatic conversion dye Sensitive assay for a short time exposure of 3–6 hours pH-dependent absorption of the dye in the viable cell matrix. Not suitable for volatile, water unstable and low solubility substances
Indirect contact test (Agar overlay), NRU	Potential cytotoxic leachates able to bind to the agar and diffuse across the plate	Suitable for investigating the high toxicity and density materials Simple and rapid for the testing of high-density materials	Unable to mimic the barrier in vivo. Some potential cytotoxic leachates are able to bind to the agar and are unable to diffuse across the plate
Tryphan blue	Membrane integrity	Easy to apply Inexpensive Widely used	Apoptosis or necrosis cannot be distinguished Limited sensitivity
Alamar blue/ Resazurin assay	Indicator of the metabolic activity	Suitable for long-term studies Highly stable in the culture medium Lower toxicity Inexpensive High sensitivity Able to monitor the cell proliferation and function of immune cells	Fluorescence interference Need long optimization procedure Can not differ cytotoxic or cytostatic
SulforhodamineB assay	Cellular protein content Cell viability Binds to protein components of cells that have been fixed on culture plates by TCA	Suitable for high-throughput screening Proper for long-term studies Highly sensitive in low cell numbers Measure total protein content and does rely on cell functionality Reproducibility Best linearity Few described interferences. Stability over time and low cost	Cannot differ living or dead cells Limited to manual or semiautomatic screening Consist of several washing step Rarely presents interferences, but evaluates the entire protein content Requiring removal of dead cells from the plate to determine cell viability

Method	Mechanism of action	Advantages	Disadvantages
Live/Dead	Cell metabolism	Proper for high-throughput studies Non-radioactive Rapid process High sensitivity, fast and simple handling	Not very sensitive in adherent cells Need higher-sensitive microscopy Nanoparticles favor PI entry and increase false positive results; higher cost than other techniques
LDH release Assay	Cell membrane integrity and cell metabolism	Widely used an accepted Absorbance or fluorescent options	Low sensitivity Not suitable for long-term studies False positive results
G6PD release Assay	Cell membrane integrity and cell metabolism	More sensitive and efficient than LDH Short-term protocol	Time-consuming Not suitable for long-term studies
ATP assay	ATP production	Very good sensitivity Short-term protocol Large usage areas	Cannot differ cytotoxic or cytostatic
Protease viability Marker assay	Differential protease activity	Excellent correlation with established methods Combatible with downstream applications Non-toxic Short incubation time Differ living or dead cells	No significant advantages
Flow cytometry	Measures optic and fluorescent characteristics of a single cell or other particles in a fluid stream as they pass through a light source	A rapid and reliable method capable of promoting quantitative evaluation of viable cells in suspension and multiple cellular processes, and assessing the type of cell death type	High cost of instruments and markers, specialists for execution is needed, limited in the analysis of tissue architecture and intercellular interactions
Clonogenic cell survival assay	Proliferation ability of the cell	Suitable for long-term cytotoxicity screening Consider reversible damage or resistance against agents	Limited dynamic range Not suitable to test the impacts of agents that do not target DNA synthesis
H3 thymidine Uptake	DNA replication	No significant advantages	Harmful effects Difficulties in handling Time-consuming
BrdU	DNA replication	Reduced equipment and time Suitable with simultaneous techniques	Harsh labeling conditions Potential carcinogen
Phospho-histone H3 detection	Cell division	All four stages of mitosis detected	Time-consuming
Raman micro Spectrometry	Interaction of electromagnetic radiation with the sample molecule	Very rapid Non-invasive No damage to the cells	No significant advantages

Table 1.
The mechanisms, advantages, and disadvantages of cytotoxicity/proliferation assays mentioned in this chapter.

used for similar applications [33]. When preparing cell cultures for MTT assays, it is important to avoid using colored additives in the culture medium, such as phenol red, as they can interfere with the development of formazan color. Additionally, the MTT assay may not be suitable for certain test substances, especially those that can directly reduce tetrazolium salts [32]. In such cases, alternative assays can be employed, such as measuring ATP levels via bioluminescence or assessing the accumulation of the supravital dye neutral red in lysosomes [34, 35].

Testing plasma membrane damage could be another key event that occurred as a consequence of the compromised cell plasma integrity, and then cytosolic compounds can freely move outside the cell into the cell culture medium. For example, LDH is a stable enzyme that leaks from the cell in relatively high amounts upon cell plasma membrane damage. It catalyzes the interconversion of pyruvate and lactate with concomitant interconversion of reduced and oxidized Nicotinamide adenine dinucleotide (NADH). The consumption of NADH can be measured spectrophotometrically, providing an indication proportional to LDH activity [36]. Other cytotoxicity methods that assess damage to the plasma membrane use reporter dyes, which enter damaged cells upon addition to the culture medium. Examples of these dyes include propidium iodide and Trypan blue [33].

Selection of exposure conditions: Assessing the cytotoxic potential of a chemical is crucial to consider the relevance of the tested concentrations. Two main factors should be addressed: the relevance of the concentrations used in the *in vitro* system and their correlation with in vivo conditions. The first factor involves understanding the biokinetics of the compound within the *in vitro* system. The actual concentration causing toxic effects is influenced not only by the initial amount added to the culture medium but also by factors such as evaporation, binding to culture devices, or interactions with medium constituents like proteins. These factors can lead to significant deviations in the actual cellular exposure concentrations, sometimes altering them by up to two orders of magnitude. This may result in a much lower free concentration in the medium and, consequently, an underestimation of the compound's cytotoxic potential [7]. The second factor is the accurate translation of *in vitro* cytotoxicity results to a risk assessment context, which involves quantitative *in vitro*-to-in vivo extrapolation. This process must account for differences in cellular exposure between the *in vitro* and in vivo environments, as well as the in vivo biokinetics of the compound [37, 38].

In case of the unavailability of prior information on the expected cytotoxic concentrations derived from structural or physico-chemical properties, it is advisable to conduct at least two rounds of testing. Each round should include three biological replicates (i.e., different cell batches) and three technical replicates (i.e., different wells on a multiwell plate). In the initial round, test a minimum of 10 concentrations across a broad range, from 1 nM to 10 mM. In the subsequent round, narrow down the concentration range, typically to the μM range, and further refine as needed in additional testing phases. Additionally, the duration of exposure is a critical factor. Some toxicological responses can lead to significant changes in gene expression within just 1 hour of exposure, with only minor variations across different concentrations [39]. However, general cytotoxicity tests often use exposure times ranging from 1 to 72 hours, and this duration may need to be optimized based on the specific testing requirements. It is also highly recommended to assess the *in vitro* biokinetics of the compound, such as by measuring the free concentration using techniques like solid-phase micro-extraction [7, 40].

Implementing an appropriate set of controls is crucial for accurately interpreting *in vitro* cytotoxicity testing results. Typically, test compounds may not be fully soluble in cell culture media and thus require the use of co-solvents like DMSO, ethanol, or methanol. While ethanol and methanol are known cytotoxicants, DMSO is often used in cell cultures, such as with hepatocytes, due to its potential benefits on cell functionality. However, DMSO can also be detrimental to cells. Therefore, including a solvent control is essential when using such organic solvents to enhance the solubility of test compounds. Additionally, a positive control, which is a compound known to activate the biomarker of interest, should be included. Tamoxifen has been demonstrated to be an effective positive control in MTT and ATP-based cytotoxicity assays [27, 32]. Compounds like sodium lauryl sulfate, which damage the cell membrane, are suitable positive controls for LDH leakage assays and reporter dye uptake tests. Negative controls, though often overlooked, are just as important as positive controls. The cell culture medium itself serves as a basic negative control, but it might be necessary to test specific chemicals as true negative controls. Additionally, care must be taken to avoid introducing mechanical stress during the addition of controls and test compounds to the culture medium or while handling cell culture plates, as this can also cause cytotoxicity. For concerns about phototoxicity or temperature instability of the test compound, specific incubation conditions may be required [41].

3. Cytotoxicity tests for cosmetic ingredients and products

The global demand for cosmetics has been escalating annually, with projections estimating the market will reach $675 billion by 2020, reflecting a compound annual growth rate of 6.4%. Skin irritants are the predominant cause of non-immunological dermatitis. Consequently, there is an increased imperative to intensify the safety assessment of cosmetic preservatives [10]. Nearly a decade past the deadline established by the 7th Amendment to the EU Cosmetics Directive, which prohibited the sale of animal-tested cosmetics from 2013, the use of animal models for cosmetic testing remains a contentious issue [9]. The testing strategy involves a combination of traditional in vivo and ex vivo assays to provide physicochemical data, in silico approaches such as quantitative structure-activity relationship (QSAR) modeling and read-across techniques, and physiologically-based toxicokinetic (PBTK) modeling. These should be integrated with *in vitro* and ex vivo methodologies using a Weight of Evidence (WoE) approach, along with historical animal data (from before the legislative ban) and, where possible, data derived from human studies, including clinical trials and biomonitoring [9, 42].

Cytotoxicity testing is a prevalent method for assessing the toxicity of cosmetic ingredients and products in preclinical studies. Typically, these assays involve incubating a reagent with a cell population, where viable cells convert a substrate into a detectable colored or fluorescent product using absorbance or colorimetric detection equipment [6, 43]. In evaluating cell viability, various methodologies are available (**Table 1**), but each generally measures only a single cell parameter, which can be limiting and prone to inaccuracies. MTT assay relies on mitochondrial activity, whereas LIVE/DEAD™ assay distinguishes between live and dead cells by using calcein-AM, which is converted into green fluorescent calcein by intracellular esterases in live cells, and ethidium homodimer-1 (EthD-1), which binds to nucleic acids in dead or membrane-damaged cells, emitting red fluorescence. This allows both qualitative and quantitative assessment of cytotoxicity [6]. In the SRB assay, sulforhodamine B (SRB) binds to the basic amino acids in proteins of viable cells during fixation. The greater the SRB binding, the lower the cytotoxicity of the test sample. Thus, choosing an appropriate cell viability assay involves considering factors such as the assay's nature and duration, detection requirements, the chemical structure of the compound, and the inherent limitations of each assay, which may result in varying quantitative outcomes [44]. The differences in methodologies used by research groups highlight the need for the development of standardized guidelines to ensure consistent and reliable results in cell viability assays.

Commercially available reconstructed human epidermis models exhibit notable similarities to natural human skin and are valuable tools for assessing the safety of pharmaceutical and cosmetic substances. Nonetheless, these models currently lack certain anatomical features, such as hair follicles, sebaceous glands, nerves, and both circulatory and lymphatic systems, which limits their similarity to in vivo conditions [10]. To assess cytotoxicity as an endpoint for cell viability and to evaluate the eye irritation potential of cosmetic preservatives, cytotoxicity assays using MTT and Neutral Red Uptake (NRU) were conducted on human keratinocytes (HaCaT), human dermal fibroblasts (HDFa), and human hepatoma cells (HepG2). The eye irritation potential was assessed using the Hen's Egg Test-Chorioallantoic Membrane (HET-CAM). The preservatives tested included methylparaben (MP), propylparaben (PP), phenoxyethanol (PE), and a combination of methylchloroisothiazolinone and methylisothiazolinone (CMI/MI). All preservatives demonstrated cytotoxic effects within the allowable concentrations for use in cosmetics. According to the HET-CAM test, PE and CMI/MI were classified as severe irritants, while MP and PP were classified as moderate and poor irritants, respectively. Comprehensive safety evaluations are essential to confirm that the benefits of preservatives in cosmetic products do not pose harmful exposure levels to consumers.

In vitro tests based on cytotoxicity and cell functionality, including those outlined in OECD guidelines, are crucial for safety assessment. Specifically, the Short Time Exposure (STE) test method, employing a rabbit corneal cell line, is used to evaluate the eye irritation potential of chemicals by measuring their cytotoxic effects [11, 45]. Reconstructed human tissue (RhT)-based testing methodologies, including several OECD guidelines, provide valuable *in vitro* assessments for chemical safety. The Reconstructed Human Cornea-like Epithelium (RhCE) test method evaluates cytotoxicity by utilizing the MTT assay [46]. This guideline incorporates High-Performance Liquid Chromatography (HPLC) or Ultra-Performance Liquid Chromatography (UPLC) techniques to measure formazan formation, addressing potential interference with MTT-formazan measurement due to direct MTT reduction or color interference. RhCE models are used to identify chemicals that do not necessitate classification and labeling for eye irritation or serious eye damage. However, these models are not designed to assess the potency of eye irritancy. Currently, four validated eye irritation test (EIT) methods utilizing commercially available RhCE models have been adopted: EpiOcular™ EIT, SkinEthic™ Human Corneal Epithelium (HCE) EIT, LabCyte CORNEA-MODEL 24 EIT, and MCTT HCE™ EIT. The SkinEthic™ HCE Time-to-Toxicity test method (SkinEthic™ HCE TTT, [47]) has recently been adopted as a stand-alone method to differentiate between chemicals that do not require classification for serious eye damage or eye irritation (No Cat.) and those that do (Cat. 2 for eye irritation and Cat. 1 for serious eye damage). This method is recommended as a full replacement for the in vivo Draize acute eye irritation test [48]. It includes two protocols: one for liquids (SkinEthic™ HCE TTL), which assesses viability at three exposure times (5, 16, and 120 minutes), and one for solids

(SkinEthic™ HCE TTS), which evaluates at two exposure times (30 and 120 minutes). The Vitrigel-EIT method [49] is an *in vitro* assay using a human corneal epithelial (hCE) model within a Collagen Vitrigel Membrane (CVM) chamber. This method predicts the eye irritation potential by analyzing the chemical's ability to damage the barrier function of the hCE model, measured by changes in TransEpithelial Electrical Resistance (TEER) over time. The Vitrigel-EIT method can identify chemicals that do not require classification and labeling for eye irritation or serious eye damage within the test's applicability domain for chemicals with a pH greater than 5.0, based on a 2.5% weight/volume (w/v) preparation.

The Neutral Red Uptake (NRU) cytotoxicity assay, utilizing BALB/c3T3 cells (3T3-NRU cytotoxicity assay), is extensively employed to evaluate cytotoxicity and has demonstrated its potential in predicting acute oral toxicity, as highlighted in prior research [50]. A validation study conducted jointly by the National Toxicology Program Interagency Center for the Validation of Alternative Toxicological Methods (NICEATM) and the EU Reference Laboratory for Alternatives to Animal Testing (EURL ECVAM) affirmed the utility of the 3T3-NRU assay for estimating the starting dose for acute oral toxicity [51, 52]. This validation led to the publication of OECD Guidance Document No. 129 in 2010, titled "Guidance Document on Using Cytotoxicity Assays to Estimate Starting Doses for Acute Oral Systemic Toxicity Tests" [53]. The document outlines a methodology for determining the starting dose for acute oral toxicity studies by predicting the LD50 from regression analysis based on the correlation between the 50% inhibitory concentration (IC50) obtained from the 3T3-NRU assay and the median lethal dose (LD50) recorded in the database. The use of the 3T3-NRU assay for predicting the starting dose has been shown to reduce the number of animals required. EURL ECVAM later conducted a follow-up validation study that confirmed the applicability of the 3T3-NRU assay for substances with LD50 values greater than 2000 mg/kg [12, 54] and published the "EURL ECVAM Recommendations on the 3T3 Neutral Red Uptake Cytotoxicity Assay for Acute Oral Toxicity Testing" in 2013 [12]. The Weight of Evidence (WoE) assessment refers to integrating the strengths and limitations of accumulated data to draw conclusions that are not evident from individual datasets [53].

4. Cytotoxicity test for biocompatibility of medical devices

Biomaterials can be categorized as inert biomaterials, bioactive biomaterials with coatings, and biodegradable biomaterials that degrade and are absorbed by the patient. The latter minimizes the drawbacks of permanent implants and eliminates the need for subsequent surgical removal, thus reducing potential complications for the patient. Biocompatibility is a crucial criterion for the clinical application of biomaterials. It denotes the capability of a biomaterial to function effectively without inducing toxic or harmful reactions in biological systems while eliciting a suitable host response. Factors affecting biocompatibility include the chemical, mechanical, and structural characteristics of the biomaterials, their interactions with the biological environment, and the methodologies used for evaluation. Biocompatibility testing is a critical component of the overall safety evaluation process for medical devices. Standard biocompatibility tests typically include cytotoxicity, irritation, and sensitization assessments, which are fundamental for nearly all medical devices conducting with surface and short periods [13, 17].

Cytocompatibility tests assess the biological reactivity of living cells to biomaterial extracts by evaluating cell viability, growth, and metabolic activity [14]. Toxic agents from biomaterials, such as metal ions, reactive chemicals, and residual monomers, can negatively impact cell functions and viability. This cellular damage can manifest as structural breakdown, changes in cell morphology, reduced cell adhesion and proliferation, decreased metabolic activity, and cell lysis [17].

Medical devices are typically evaluated through extract testing, which involves immersing the device or its components in a suitable extraction solvent, such as physiological saline, vegetable oil, or cell culture medium, under defined conditions. This procedure is a standard practice for assessing the biocompatibility of medical devices by measuring the potential release of substances that could interact with biological systems. Comprehensive guidelines for extract preparation are outlined in ISO 10993-12 [15]. Despite these guidelines providing detailed instructions on sample selection, preparation, experimental controls, reference materials, and extraction methods, variations in interpretation by Contract Research Organizations (CROs) may lead to inconsistencies in the results. Standardization and harmonization in the methodology for preparing extracts from medical devices are still lacking. Recent research assessing the variability in cytotoxicity methods according to ISO 10993-5:2009 [16] has underscored the significant influence of the extraction solution whether it is a medium with or without serum on test results. Even small changes in the protocol can markedly affect the predicted cytotoxicity outcomes [55]. Prior to conducting biocompatibility assessments, biomaterials derived from the final configuration of a medical device are subjected to extraction processes using semi-physiological media, such as saline solution, cottonseed oil, sesame oil, or cell culture medium, placed in small containers [17]. The extraction is typically performed through incubation for 24–72 hours at 37°C. Following this period, the resultant extract solutions are transferred into sterile glass tubes for subsequent biological testing [56]. Variability in extraction procedures, including the choice of extraction medium, can impact the relevance to in vivo conditions and the efficiency of solubilizing organic hydrophobic compounds. Utilizing an extraction vehicle containing low concentrations of dimethyl sulfoxide (less than 0.5%) can enhance the solubilization of both hydrophilic and hydrophobic substances [14]. There is a pressing need for more detailed guidance on handling materials that absorb solvents, as such interactions can alter the osmolarity of cell culture media, potentially compromising cell line viability. Testing materials with poor solubility in submerged cell cultures presents technical challenges and may result in false-negative outcomes. To address these challenges, 3D epithelial tissue models offer a promising alternative. These models can accommodate materials extracted in both polar and non-polar solvents, providing a more adaptable and potentially precise testing environment. The development and adoption of these advanced models could significantly improve the reliability of cytotoxicity evaluations for medical devices, especially those containing low-level toxic components that exhibit poor solubility in polar solvents. This approach would ensure a more accurate prediction of long-term safety and efficacy, thereby aligning *in vitro* testing more closely with actual usage scenarios of medical devices.

ISO 10993-5 outlines specific methodologies and protocols for performing cytotoxicity testing, which typically involves exposing cultured mammalian cells to extracts derived from medical devices or their materials for approximately 24 hours. Commonly employed cell lines in these assays include Balb/3T3 (fibroblasts), L929 (fibroblasts), and Vero (kidney-derived epithelial cells). Cytotoxicity testing assesses several endpoints, including cell viability, morphological changes, cell detachment, and cell lysis, to evaluate cell viability and adverse cellular responses.

ISO 10993-5 outlines three primary cytotoxicity testing methods: extract, direct contact, and indirect contact tests, which include agar overlay assays and filter diffusion assays [57]. Generally, the extract test is employed to assess the toxicity of soluble substances from medical devices and often aligns with findings from animal toxicity studies. The direct contact assay is noted for its heightened sensitivity, capable of detecting even minimal cytotoxic effects of medical devices. The agar overlay assay is appropriate for evaluating devices with substantial toxicity and bulk characteristics, while the molecular filtration method is suited for assessing the biocompatibility of low molecular weight toxic components in medical devices [17].

The cytotoxicity elution test, also known as the MEM elution test, is an *in vitro* qualitative assay used to evaluate the cytotoxicity of materials. In this test, L929 mouse fibroblast cells are incubated with an extract of the test material for 48 hours. Post-incubation, the cells are examined microscopically to assess morphological changes. The cellular responses are categorized on a scale from 0 to 4, with a grade of 2 or below (mild reactivity) indicating that the biomaterial is considered biocompatible [56]. A material is deemed cytocompatible if at least 70% of the cells remain viable [56, 58]. While the MTT assay is considered a benchmark for cytotoxicity testing, it has notable drawbacks. Variables such as cell culture conditions can influence MTT metabolism and reduction rates, and interactions between the test material and MTT may alter the assay results. For example, carbon nanotubes and calcium phosphate scaffolds can reduce MTT, and carbon nanotubes may bind the resultant formazan, affecting the test's accuracy [14, 58]. The agar overlay assay is a qualitative technique for assessing cytotoxicity through indirect contact. In this assay, subconfluent cell cultures (e.g., mouse fibroblasts L929, NIH 3T3) are covered with an agar layer. The test material is then placed on the agar and incubated for 24–72 hours. Following this exposure period, the test material is removed, and the cells underneath and surrounding the material are subjected to neutral red staining. This staining allows for semi-quantitative assessment of cellular detachment, vacuolization, and lysis. Only viable cells retain the neutral red dye, appearing red under a light microscope. This assay is particularly suitable for evaluating high-density biomaterials but is limited to assessing acute cytotoxicity due to the brief exposure period [17].

Cytotoxicity is generally classified into four categories based on specific endpoints: non-cytotoxic, mildly cytotoxic, moderately cytotoxic, and highly cytotoxic [13]. To quantify cell viability in these categories, several methodologies are frequently employed, including MTT, XTT, and neutral red uptake. Less commonly used techniques include Bradford protein assay, crystal violet staining, resazurin dye assay, and trypan blue exclusion assay. Nevertheless, there is no standardized protocol for cytotoxicity testing, and each method has its limitations. The xCELLigence real-time cell analysis (RTCA) system represents an advanced impedance-based sensor technology. This system utilizes a microelectronic sensor chip integrated into the base of the cell culture plate to provide continuous, dynamic, and quantitative monitoring of cell morphology, proliferation, and differentiation. Variations in electrode interface impedance, caused by cells adhering to the microelectrode surface, are correlated with real-time cellular conditions, allowing for the assessment of cell growth, morphology, and viability through dynamic impedance measurements [59].

5. Cytotoxicity test for nanoparticle safety assessment

In contemporary times, nanomaterials (NMs) are extensively integrated into various aspects of daily life due to their considerable advantages, as evidenced by their utilization across numerous domains, including biomedicine, engineering, food technology, cosmetics, sensing, and energy production [18]. Nonetheless, the escalating production of NMs increases the likelihood of their environmental release, resulting in unavoidable human exposure. The potential toxicity or impact of nanoparticles (NPs) on both the environment and human health can be initially evaluated *in vitro* using cellular models. However, traditional cytotoxicity assays, such as the MTT assay, have limitations, including the potential for interference from the nanoparticles being studied. To evaluate the cytotoxicity of nanoparticles (NPs), a range of conventional assays and biomarkers are employed. For instance, cell viability and proliferation can be assessed using tetrazolium-based assays such as MTT, MTS, and WST-1, as well as neutral red uptake, trypan blue exclusion, lactate dehydrogenase (LDH) release, mitochondrial membrane potential (MMP) measurement, and Alamar Blue (resazurin) assays. Alternatively, the inflammatory response of cells can be gauged by quantifying inflammatory cytokines such as IL-8, IL-6, and tumor necrosis factor through enzyme-linked immunosorbent assays (ELISA). Furthermore, the integrity of cell membranes can be evaluated using LDH release and trypan blue exclusion assays, while cell metabolism is often monitored with the Alamar Blue assay. Despite their utility in providing general information on NP cytotoxicity, these assays do not elucidate the molecular mechanisms underlying cytotoxic effects [60, 61].

The cytotoxicity of NPs generally arises from their intracellular presence [61]. However, many biomedical applications require NPs to penetrate cells to achieve their therapeutic objectives. Therefore, understanding the cellular uptake mechanisms of NPs is crucial for elucidating their cytotoxicity mechanisms and designing environmentally safer NMs with improved cellular targeting and uptake characteristics for therapeutic use. When NPs are introduced into biological fluids, they encounter a different medium compared to their synthesis environment, potentially altering their physical and chemical properties. To stabilize themselves, NPs often adsorb surrounding biomolecules (such as proteins and lipids), forming a biomolecular or protein corona, which may modify their identity [62]. The physicochemical properties of NPs, including size, shape, surface functionalization, surface chemistry, chemical composition, and concentration, play a critical role in their design for biomedical and other applications. These properties can significantly influence interactions at the bionano interface, thereby affecting cellular uptake and the resultant nanotoxicity of the NPs.

Size: The dimension of nanoparticles (NPs) significantly impacts their cellular uptake and cytotoxicity. Smaller NPs (based on primary size rather than hydrodynamic size) of both TiO_2 and Al_2O_3 exhibit increased cytotoxicity and a more substantial reduction in cellular metabolic activity [60]. The relationship between NP size and interaction with cell membranes reveals that larger NPs (>60 nm) may experience steric hindrance, impeding their ability to interact with cell membranes. Conversely, NPs smaller than the receptor diffusion cutoff (<30 nm) might not recruit a sufficient number of cell membrane receptors in the interaction zone to overcome the elastic recoil force, thereby hindering membrane wrapping [63]. Generally, smaller-sized NPs are associated with enhanced cellular uptake and increased cytotoxicity. Due to their diminutive size, nanoparticles can easily diffuse through the gastrointestinal tract or the gill membranes of aquatic organisms. Additionally, nanoparticle dimensions are critical in determining their aggregation patterns within the human body and other organisms. For instance, a review by Dong et al. analyzed 76 selected studies on the size-dependent cytotoxicity of amorphous silica NPs ($aSiO_2$ NPs) and found that 76% of these studies reported greater cytotoxicity for smaller-sized $aSiO_2$ NPs. However, it is crucial to consider cell type variations, as cytotoxicity depends on the predominant cellular uptake pathways in different cell types [64]. In some cases, increased cellular uptake of NPs correlates with greater cytotoxicity [65]. However, there are exceptions where NP cytotoxicity is not directly proportional to cellular uptake. In such instances, factors like NP surface area, instability, and ion release contribute to cytotoxic effects rather than the quantity of the toxicant.

Shape: The shape of NPs can be tailored through adjustments in experimental conditions during synthesis, such as supersaturation, reducing agents, temperature, surfactants, and secondary nucleation. NPs can assume various shapes and geometries, including spherical, rod-like, flower-like, star-shaped, disk-like, cubic, prismatic, and needle-like forms. Gold nanoparticles (AuNPs) are prevalent in biomedical applications, and numerous studies have explored the impact of NP shape on cellular uptake and cytotoxicity. For example, Woźniak et al. [66] compared the *in vitro* cytotoxicity of differently shaped and sized bare (non-coated) AuNPs in cancer (HeLa) and normal (HEK293T) cell lines, revealing that Au nanospheres (AuNS) and Au nanorods (AuNRs) exhibited higher cytotoxicity compared to star-, flower-, and prism-shaped AuNPs.

Surface charge: The surface charge of nanoparticles (NPs) can significantly influence their interactions with cell membranes, the formation of a protein corona, and, consequently, the extent of cellular uptake. Geiser et al. [67] observed that particles can penetrate into the epithelial lining after entering the small airways and alveoli, and that surface reactivity can modify the biological effects of the particles. For example, surface modifications of silica nanoparticles can impact their inflammatory potential, fibrogenic properties, and cytotoxicity [67]. Research has demonstrated that positively charged nanoparticles are more readily internalized by cells compared to negatively charged or neutral nanoparticles. Furthermore, positively charged nanoparticles can bind to negatively charged DNA, potentially causing genetic damage, which contributes to their increased toxicity [68]. Variations in the surface chemistry of nanoparticles have been shown to result in different toxicity profiles depending on the nanoparticle type. Generally, charged nanoparticles exhibit higher cellular uptake compared to neutral nanoparticles [63]. Given that cell membranes are negatively charged due to the anionic phospholipid head groups and certain carbohydrates like sialic acid, cationic nanoparticles tend to be more readily taken up by non-phagocytic cells compared to anionic nanoparticles. However, in some cases, anionic nanoparticles may exhibit higher cellular uptake in phagocytic cells [69]. Additionally, the surface charge of nanoparticles can influence their cellular uptake pathways. Surface functionalization of nanoparticles, which involves modifying the surface ligands, primarily affects parameters such as surface charge and hydrophobicity, thereby influencing the protein core, cellular uptake, and cytotoxicity of the nanoparticles. Specific surface functionalities can also be employed to enhance targeting capabilities.

Cell viability responses to nanoparticles are cell line-dependent. A549 cells (a lung epithelial cell line) are more sensitive to nanoparticles compared to HepG2 cells (a liver cell line). This increased sensitivity in A549 cells is consistent with their respiratory epithelial nature, making them more responsive to particulate exposure compared to HepG2 cells, which are adapted to handle toxic substances. This observation is supported by studies showing that A549 cells exhibit higher oxidative stress, lactate dehydrogenase leakage, decreased glutathione levels, mitochondrial membrane potential dissipation, increased apoptotic gene expression, and reduced cellular viability upon exposure to $CuFe_2O_4$ and $ZnFe_2O_4$ nanoparticles [70, 71]. In contrast, HepG2 cells show lower susceptibility and a less toxic response to various sizes and concentrations of silica nanoparticles, including lower reactive oxygen species (ROS) generation, reduced glutathione depletion, and less decline in cell viability [72]. Additionally, A549 cells exhibit more significant mitochondrial membrane potential reduction and lower viability when exposed to silver nanoparticles compared to HepG2 cells. This discrepancy in cytotoxic responses may be attributed to the liver's superior detoxification capacity, facilitated by its phase I and II enzymatic systems, compared to the lung.

A significant mechanism contributing to nanoparticle toxicity is their cytotoxicity, which is influenced by the quality of the nanoparticles, their deposition sites, and the mode of administration [19]. Sohaebuddin et al. [73] reported that titanium dioxide (TiO_2) and silicon dioxide (SiO_2) nanoparticles induced cytotoxic effects in three different cell lines: RAW 264.7 macrophages, telomerase-immortalized bronchiolar epithelial cells, and 3T3 fibroblasts. They concluded that the extent of toxicity and intracellular responses are dependent on both the concentration and size of the nanoparticles. Patra et al. [74] found that the toxicity of gold nanoparticles was contingent on the type of cell line and the physical and chemical properties of the nanoparticles. Variability in toxicity was also observed between human lung and liver cancer cell lines [75]. Huang et al. [76] reported that zinc oxide nanoparticles exert significant toxic effects on both bacterial and mammalian cells. Common toxic outcomes of zinc-based nanoparticles include damage to cell membranes and elevated oxidative stress. These findings suggest that nanoparticles can act as potent cytotoxins. The studies indicate that the generation of reactive oxygen species (ROS) and resulting cytotoxicity may be key mechanisms underlying the adverse effects of nanomaterials, including damage to DNA and cell membranes. While extensive research has been conducted to elucidate the mechanisms of nanoparticle toxicity, further understanding is necessary to mitigate the toxicological side effects associated with these materials.

6. Conclusion

The evaluation of efficacy and safety is a fundamental prerequisite before the introduction of new chemicals, therapeutic agents, cosmetics, biomaterials, medical devices, and nanoparticles. In pharmaceutical research, cytotoxicity tests are employed to screen novel drug candidates at an early stage, identifying potential harmful effects to prevent adverse reactions later in the development process. Cytotoxicity assays are crucial for determining the dose-response relationship of a drug and establishing the concentration at which it becomes toxic to cells. This information is essential for defining safe dosage levels for further testing and eventual clinical use. Additionally, cytotoxicity assays provide insights into the mechanisms through which a drug induces cell death or damage, aiding in the prediction of potential side effects and guiding modifications to improve safety. When combined with other *in vitro* and in vivo tests, cytotoxicity assays contribute to a comprehensive preclinical safety evaluation, helping to identify and mitigate risks before clinical trials. These assays also allow researchers to compare the safety profiles of new drugs with existing treatments, facilitating a comparative analysis that can highlight potential advantages or disadvantages of new compounds. Regulatory agencies require extensive safety data, including cytotoxicity results, before approving new drugs for clinical trials and market release. The certification of cosmetics and medical devices also requires approval of a safety profile obtained from toxicity and biocompatibility testing.

Cytotoxicity testing is also a prevalent method for assessing the toxicity of cosmetic ingredients and products in preclinical studies. Commercially available reconstructed human epidermis models, which exhibit notable similarities to natural human skin, serve as valuable tools for assessing the safety of pharmaceutical and cosmetic substances. *In vitro* tests based on cytotoxicity and cell functionality, including those outlined in OECD guidelines, are critical for safety assessment. For example, the Short Time Exposure (STE) test method, which employs a rabbit corneal cell line, is used to evaluate the eye irritation potential of chemicals by measuring their cytotoxic effects.

Biocompatibility testing is an integral component of the overall safety evaluation process for medical devices. Standard biocompatibility tests typically include assessments of cytotoxicity, irritation, and sensitization, which are fundamental for nearly all medical devices that come into contact with surfaces or are used for short periods. Cytocompatibility tests assess the biological reactivity of living cells to biomaterial extracts by evaluating parameters such as cell viability, growth, and metabolic activity.

Nanomaterials (NMs) are increasingly integrated into various aspects of daily life due to their significant advantages, as evidenced by their use across numerous domains, including biomedicine, engineering, food technology, cosmetics, and energy production. However, the escalating production of NMs increases the likelihood of environmental release, leading to unavoidable human exposure. The potential toxicity or impact of nanoparticles (NPs) on both the environment and human health can be initially evaluated *in vitro* using cellular models. Nevertheless, traditional cytotoxicity assays have limitations, including the potential for interference from the nanoparticles being studied. The physicochemical properties of NPs, including size, shape, surface functionalization, surface chemistry, chemical composition, and concentration, are critical in their design for biomedical and other applications. These properties significantly influence interactions at the bionano interface, thereby affecting cellular uptake and the resultant nanotoxicity of the NPs.

Overall, there are a number of available existing cytotoxicity assays; however, testing strategy and methodology need to be validated. This chapter provides an overview of the key concepts and methods in cytotoxicity testing, highlighting its importance across various fields and the ongoing advancements in this critical area of research.

Conflict of interest

The authors declare no conflict of interest.

Author details

Yüksel Çetin
The Scientific and Technological Research Council of Turkey (TUBITAK), Marmara Research Center (MAM), Life Sciences Medical Biotechnology, Gebze, Kocaeli, Turkey

*Address all correspondence to: yuksel.cetin@tubitak.gov.tr

References

[1] Vinken M, Blaauboer BJ. In vitro testing of basal cytotoxicity: Establishment of an adverse outcome pathway from chemical insult to cell death. Toxicology In Vitro. 2017;**39**: 104-110. DOI: 10.1016/j.tiv.2016.12.004

[2] Fraczek J et al. Primary hepatocyte cultures for pharmaco-toxicological studies: At the busy crossroad of various anti-dedifferentiation strategies. Archives of Toxicology. 2013;**87**:577-610. DOI: 10.1007/s00204-012-0983-3

[3] Vinken M, Vanhaecke T, Rogiers V. Primary hepatocyte cultures as in vitro tools for toxicity testing: Quo vadis? Toxicology In Vitro. 2012;**26**(3):541-544. DOI: 10.1016/j.tiv.2012.01.002

[4] Adan A, Kiraz Y, Baran Y. Cell proliferation and cytotoxicity assays. Current Pharmaceutical Biotechnology. 2016;**17**(14):1213-1221. DOI: 10.2174/138 9201017666160808160513

[5] Sukumaran A et al. Cytotoxicity and cell viability assessment of biomaterials. In: Cytotoxicity-Understanding Cellular Damage and Response. IntechOpen; 2023

[6] Nabarretti BH et al. A review of alternative methods to the use of animals in safety evaluation of cosmetics. einstein (Sao Paulo). 2022;**20**:eRB5578. DOI: 10.31744/einstein_journal/2022RB5578

[7] Kramer NI, Van Eijkeren JC, Hermens JL. Influence of albumin on sorption kinetics in solid-phase microextraction: Consequences for chemical analyses and uptake processes. Analytical Chemistry. 2007;**79**(18):6941-6948. DOI: 10.1021/ac070574n

[8] Zhang Q et al. Bridging the data gap from in vitro toxicity testing to chemical safety assessment through computational modeling. Frontiers in Public Health. 2018;**6**:261. DOI: 10.3389/fpubh.2018.00261

[9] Silva RJ, Tamburic S. A state-of-the-art review on the alternatives to animal testing for the safety assessment of cosmetics. Cosmetics. 2022;**9**(5):90. DOI: 10.3390/cosmetics9050090

[10] Corrêa GdOP et al. In vitro evaluation of the cytotoxicity and eye irritation potential of preservatives widely used in cosmetics. Brazilian. Journal of Pharmaceutical Sciences. 2022;**58**:e20039. DOI: 10.1590/s2175-97902022e20039

[11] Bernauer U et al. The SCCS Notes of Guidance for the Testing of Cosmetic Ingredients and Their Safety Evaluation-12th Revision-SCCS/1647/22. Luxembourg: Commission Européenne; 2023

[12] Prieto PMDP et al. EURL ECVAM Recommendation on the 3T3 Neutral Red Uptake Cytotoxicity Assay for Acute Oral Toxicity Testing. Luxembourg: European Commission; 2013

[13] Kandárová H, Pôbiš P. The "Big Three" in biocompatibility testing of medical devices: Implementation of alternatives to animal experimentation—Are we there yet? Frontiers in Toxicology. 2024;**5**:1337468. DOI: 10.3389/ftox.2023.1337468

[14] Bruinink A, Luginbuehl R. Evaluation of biocompatibility using in vitro methods: Interpretation and limitations. In: Tissue Engineering III: Cell-Surface Interactions for Tissue Culture. Luxembourg: European Commission; 2012. pp. 117-152. DOI: 10.1007/10_2011_111

[15] ISO 10993-12:2021. Biological Evaluation of Medical Devices Part 12: Sample Preparation and Reference Materials. 5th ed. Geneva: International Organization for Standardization; 2021

[16] The International Organization for Standardization/Technical Committee 194. Biological Evaluation of Medical Devices Part 5: Tests for in Vitro Cytotoxicity. 3rd ed. Geneva; 2009

[17] Huzum B et al. Biocompatibility assessment of biomaterials used in orthopedic devices: An overview. Experimental and Therapeutic Medicine. 2021;**22**(5):1-9. DOI: 10.3892/etm.2021.10750

[18] Awashra M, Młynarz P. The toxicity of nanoparticles and their interaction with cells: An in vitro metabolomic perspective. Nanoscale Advances. 2023;**5**(10):2674-2723. DOI: 10.1039/d2na00534d

[19] Li X et al. Biocompatibility and toxicity of nanoparticles and nanotubes. Journal of Nanomaterials. 2012;**2012**(1):548389. DOI: 10.1155/2012/548389

[20] Gennari A et al. Strategies to replace in vivo acute systemic toxicity testing: The report and recommendations of ECVAM workshop 50. Alternatives to Laboratory Animals. 2004;**32**(4):437-459. DOI: 10.1177/026119290403200417

[21] Schoonen W, Westerink W, Horbach GJ. High-throughput screening for analysis of in vitro toxicity. EXS. 2009;**99**(99):401-521

[22] Houck KA, Kavlock RJ. Understanding mechanisms of toxicity: Insights from drug discovery research. Toxicology and Applied Pharmacology. 2008;**227**(2):163-178. DOI: 10.1016/j.taap.2007.10.022

[23] Escher BI et al. Baseline toxicity (narcosis) of organic chemicals determined by in vitro membrane potential measurements in energy-transducing membranes. Environmental Science & Technology. 2002;**36**(9):1971-1979. DOI: 10.1021/es015844c

[24] Eisenbrand G et al. Methods of in vitro toxicology. Food and Chemical Toxicology. 2002;**40**(2-3):193-236. DOI: 10.1016/S0278-6915(01)00118-1

[25] Jones DP et al. Mechanisms of pathogenesis in drug hepatotoxicity putting the stress on mitochondria. Molecular Interventions. 2010;**10**(2):98. DOI: 10.1124/mi.10.2.7

[26] Pessayre D et al. Mitochondrial involvement in drug-induced liver injury. Adverse drug reactions. Handbook of Experimental Pharmacology. 2010;**196**:311-365. DOI: 10.1007/978-3-642-00663-0_11

[27] Shukla SJ et al. The future of toxicity testing: A focus on in vitro methods using a quantitative high-throughput screening platform. Drug Discovery Today. 2010;**15**(23-24):997-1007. DOI: 10.1016/j.drudis.2010.07.007

[28] Qiao L, Farrell GC. The effects of cell density, attachment substratum and dexamethasone on spontaneous apoptosis of rat hepatocytes in primary culture. In Vitro Cellular and Developmental Biology - Animal. 1999;**35**:417-424. DOI: 10.1007/s11626-999-0117-2

[29] Vanhaecke T et al. Effect of the histone deacetylase inhibitor trichostatin A on spontaneous apoptosis in various types of adult rat hepatocyte cultures. Biochemical Pharmacology. 2004;**68**(4):753-760. DOI: 10.1016/j.bcp.2004.05.022

[30] Tuschl G et al. Serum-free collagen sandwich cultures of adult rat hepatocytes maintain liver-like properties long term: A valuable model for in vitro toxicity and drug–drug interaction studies. Chemico-Biological Interactions. 2009;**181**(1):124-137. DOI: 10.1016/j.cbi.2009.05.015

[31] Mosmann T. Rapid colorimetric assay for cellular growth and survival: Application to proliferation and cytotoxicity assays. Journal of Immunological Methods. 1983;**65**(1-2):55-63. DOI: 10.1016/0022-1759(83)90303-4

[32] Tolosa L, Donato MT, Gómez-Lechón MJ. General cytotoxicity assessment by means of the MTT assay. Protocols in in vitro hepatocyte research. Methods in Molecular Biology. 2015:333-348. DOI: 10.1007/978-1-4939-2074-7_26

[33] Gomez-Lechon M et al. In vitro evaluation of potential hepatotoxicity induced by drugs. Current Pharmaceutical Design. 2010;**16**(17):1963-1977. DOI: 10.2174/138161210791208910

[34] Babich H, Borenfreund E. Structure-activity relationship (SAR) models established in vitro with the neutral red cytotoxicity assay. Toxicology In Vitro. 1987;**1**(1):3-9. DOI: 10.1016/0887-2333(87)90031-2

[35] Fotakis G, Timbrell JA. In vitro cytotoxicity assays: Comparison of LDH, neutral red, MTT and protein assay in hepatoma cell lines following exposure to cadmium chloride. Toxicology Letters. 2006;**160**(2):171-177. DOI: 10.1016/j.toxlet.2005.07.001

[36] Bergmeyer H-U. Methods of Enzymatic Analysis. 2nd ed. New York: Academic Press; 2012. DOI: 10.1016/B978-0-12-395630-9.X5001-4

[37] Blaauboer B et al. The use of biomarkers of toxicity for integrating in vitro hazard estimates into risk assessment for humans. ALTEX. 2012;**29**(4):411-425. DOI: 10.14573/altex.2012.4.411

[38] Yoon M, Blaauboer BJ, Clewell HJ. Quantitative in vitro to in vivo extrapolation (QIVIVE): An essential element for in vitro-based risk assessment. Toxicology. 2015;**332**:1-3. DOI: 10.1016/j.tox.2015.02.002

[39] Shinde V et al. Transcriptomics of hepatocytes treated with toxicants for investigating molecular mechanisms underlying hepatotoxicity. Protocols in in vitro hepatocyte research. Methods in Molecular Biology. 2015:225-240. DOI: 10.1007/978-1-4939-2074-7_16

[40] Vaes WH et al. Solid phase microextraction as a tool to determine membrane/water partition coefficients and bioavailable concentrations in in vitro systems. Chemical Research in Toxicology. 1997;**10**(10):1067-1072. DOI: 10.1021/tx970109t

[41] Cooper-Hannan R, Harbell JW, Coecke S, Balls M, Bowe G, Cervinka M, et al. The principles of good laboratory practice: Application to in vitro toxicology studies. Alternatives to Laboratory Animals. 1999;**27**:539-577

[42] Rogiers V et al. The way forward for assessing the human health safety of cosmetics in the EU-workshop proceedings. Toxicology. 2020;**436**:152421. DOI: 10.1016/j.tox.2020.152421

[43] Riss TL et al. Cell viability assays. In: Assay Guidance Manual. Bethesda (MD): Eli Lilly & Company and the National Center for Advancing Translational Sciences; 2016

[44] Burga-Sánchez J. Efeito Citotóxico e Anti-Inflamatório da Articaína-2-Hidroxipropil-Beta-Ciclodextrina Sobre Células Escamosas de Carcinoma de Língua. 2018

[45] OECD Test Guideline No. 491. Short Time Exposure In Vitro Test Method for Identifying (i) Chemicals Inducing Serious Eye Damage and (ii) Chemicals Not Requiring Classification for Eye Irritation or Serious Eye Damage. Paris: Organisation for Economic Cooperation and Development; 2020

[46] OECD Test Guideline No. 492. Reconstructed Human Cornea-Like Epithelium (RhCE) Test Method for Identifying Chemicals Not Requiring Classification and Labelling for Eye Irritation or Serious Eye Damage. Paris: Organisation for Economic Cooperation and Development; 2019

[47] OECD Test Guideline No. 492B. Reconstructed Human Cornea-Like Epithelium (RHCE) Test Method for Eye Hazard Identification. Paris: Organisation for Economic Cooperation and Development; 2022

[48] OECD Test Guideline No. 492B. Acute Eye Irritation/Corrosion. Paris: Organisation for Economic Cooperation and Development; 2021

[49] OECD Test Guideline No. 492B. Vitrigel-Eye Irritancy Test Method for Identifying Chemicals Not Requiring Classification and Labelling for Eye Irritation or Serious Eye Damage. Paris: Organisation for Economic Cooperation and Development; 2021

[50] Halle W et al. The registry of cytotoxicity: Toxicity testing in cell cultures to predict acute toxicity (LD50) and to reduce testing in animals. Alternatives to Laboratory Animals. 2003;**31**(2):89-89. DOI: 10.1177/026119290303100204

[51] NICEATM N. Background Review Document: In Vitro Cytotoxicity Test Methods for Estimating Acute Oral Systemic Toxicity. NIH Publication No. 01-4499. Research Triangle Park, NC: National Institute for Environmental Health Sciences. 2006. Available from: http://iccvam.niehs.nih.gov/

[52] ICCVAM N. ICCVAM Test Method Evaluation Report: In Vitro Cytotoxicity Test Methods for Estimating Starting Doses for Acute Oral Systemic Toxicity Testing. NIH Publication No. 01-4499. Research Triangle Park, NC: National Institute for Environmental Health Sciences. 2006. Available from: http://iccvam.niehs.nih.gov/

[53] OECD. Guidance document on using cytotoxicity tests to estimate starting doses for acute oral systemic toxicity tests. In: Series on Testing and Assessment No. 129. Paris: Organisation for Economic Cooperation and Development; 2010

[54] ECVAM. Follow-up Study on the Predictive Capacity of the 3T3 Neutral Red Uptake Cytotoxicity Assay to Correctly Identify Substances Not Classified for Acute Oral Toxicity Under the EU CLP System (LD50 > 2000 mg/kg), Final Study Report. Luxembourg: European Commission; 2011

[55] Jablonská E et al. Test conditions can significantly affect the results of in vitro cytotoxicity testing of degradable metallic biomaterials. Scientific Reports. 2021;**11**(1):6628. DOI: 10.1038/s41598-021-85019-6

[56] Assad M, Jackson N. Biocompatibility evaluation of orthopedic biomaterials and medical devices: A review of safety and efficacy models. In: Reference Module in Biomedical Sciences. Encyclopedia of Biomedical Engineering; 2019. pp. 281-309. DOI: 10.1016/B978-0-12-801238-3.11104-3

[57] Li W, Zhou J, Xu Y. Study of the in vitro cytotoxicity testing of medical devices. Biomedical Reports. 2015;**3**(5):617-620. DOI: 10.3892/br.2015.481

[58] Iqbal H, Keshavarz T. The challenge of biocompatibility evaluation of biocomposites. In: Biomedical Composites. Elsevier; 2017. pp. 303-334

[59] Ke N et al. The xCELLigence system for real-time and label-free monitoring of cell viability. Mammalian cell viability: Methods and protocols. Methods in Molecular Biology. 2011;**740**:33-43

[60] Wei Z et al. Effect of particle size on in vitro cytotoxicity of titania and alumina nanoparticles. Journal of Experimental Nanoscience. 2014;**9**(6):625-638

[61] Klassen A et al. Metabolomics: Definitions and significance in systems biology. Metabolomics: From fundamentals to clinical applications. Advances in Experimental Medicine and Biology. 2017;**965**:3-17. DOI: 10.1007/978-3-319-47656-8_1

[62] Nierenberg D, Khaled AR, Flores O. Formation of a protein corona influences the biological identity of nanomaterials. Reports of Practical Oncology and Radiotherapy. 2018;**23**(4):300-308. DOI: 10.1016/j.rpor.2018.05.005

[63] Kettler K et al. Cellular uptake of nanoparticles as determined by particle properties, experimental conditions, and cell type. Environmental Toxicology and Chemistry. 2014;**33**(3):481-492. DOI: 10.1002/etc.2470

[64] Chithrani BD, Chan WC. Elucidating the mechanism of cellular uptake and removal of protein-coated gold nanoparticles of different sizes and shapes. Nano Letters. 2007;**7**(6): 1542-1550. DOI: 10.1021/nl070363y

[65] Sun H et al. Cytotoxicity-related bioeffects induced by nanoparticles: The role of surface chemistry. Frontiers in Bioengineering and Biotechnology. 2019;**7**:414. DOI: 10.3389/fbioe.2019.00414

[66] Woźniak A et al. Size and shape-dependent cytotoxicity profile of gold nanoparticles for biomedical applications. Journal of Materials Science: Materials in Medicine. 2017;**28**: 1-11. DOI: 10.1007/s10856-017-5902-y

[67] Geiser M, Schurch S, Gehr P. Influence of surface chemistry and topography of particles on their immersion into the lung's surface-lining layer. Journal of Applied Physiology. 2003;**94**:1793-1801. DOI: 10.1152/japplphysiol.00514.2002

[68] Liu Y et al. Intracellular dynamics of cationic and anionic polystyrene nanoparticles without direct interaction with mitotic spindle and chromosomes. Biomaterials. 2011;**32**(32):8291-8303. DOI: 10.1016/j.biomaterials.2011.07.037

[69] Fröhlich E. The role of surface charge in cellular uptake and cytotoxicity of medical nanoparticles. International Journal of Nanomedicine. 2012;**7**: 5577-5591. DOI: 10.2147/IJN.S36111

[70] Alhadlaq HA, Akhtar MJ, Ahamed M. Zinc ferrite nanoparticle-induced cytotoxicity and oxidative stress in different human cells. Cell & Bioscience. 2015;**5**:1-11

[71] Ahmad J et al. Differential cytotoxicity of copper ferrite nanoparticles in different human cells. Journal of Applied Toxicology. 2016;**36**(10):1284-1293. DOI: 10.1002/jat.3299

[72] Kim I-Y et al. Toxicity of silica nanoparticles depends on size, dose, and cell type. Nanomedicine: Nanotechnology, Biology and Medicine. 2015;**11**(6):1407-1416. DOI: 10.1016/j.nano.2015.03.004

[73] Sohaebuddin SK, Thevenot PT, Baker D, Eaton JW, Tang L. Nanomaterial cytotoxicity is composition, size, and cell type dependent. Part. Fibre Toxicology. 2010;**7**:1-17. DOI: 10.1186/1743-8977-7-22

[74] Patra HK et al. Cell selective response to gold nanoparticles. Nanomedicine: Nanotechnology, Biology and Medicine. 2007;**3**(2):111-119. DOI: 10.1016/j.nano.2007.03.005

[75] Schiewe MH et al. Use of a bacterial bioluminescence assay to assess toxicity of contaminated marine sediments. Canadian Journal of Fisheries and Aquatic Sciences. 1985;**42**(7):1244-1248. DOI: 10.1139/f85-154

[76] Huang Z et al. Toxicological effect of ZnO nanoparticles based on bacteria. Langmuir. 2008;**24**(8):4140-4144. DOI: 10.1021/la7035949

Chapter 3

In Vitro Cytotoxicity Determination: Avoiding Pitfalls

Mashilo Matotoka and Peter Masoko

Abstract

In vitro cytotoxicity assays are critical tools for assessing the potential toxicity of compounds in early-stage drug discovery, toxicology, and biomedical research. These assays help evaluate the effects of chemical, pharmaceutical, and biological agents on cellular health and viability. However, the reliability of cytotoxicity data is often compromised by a variety of experimental pitfalls. This chapter discusses the key factors that can lead to inaccurate or misleading results in cytotoxicity assays and provides guidelines for avoiding them. Common issues such as inappropriate assay selection, interference from serum components like fetal bovine serum (FBS), cell density variations, and incorrect incubation times are highlighted. The importance of using appropriate controls, avoiding solvent-induced toxicity, and preventing compound aggregation is also emphasized. By optimizing experimental conditions and understanding the limitations of each assay type, researchers can enhance the precision of their *in vitro* cytotoxicity tests. This chapter aims to provide a comprehensive guide to improving experimental design, ensuring reproducibility, and generating reliable data that can be confidently applied in drug development and toxicological evaluations.

Keywords: cytotoxicity, cell lines, assay methods, standardization, optimization

1. Introduction

Cytotoxicity refers to a substance's ability to cause damage or death to cells, which is crucial for understanding how harmful a substance might be, especially for medical treatments or devices [1–4]. *In vitro* cytotoxicity testing is a laboratory technique used to assess the potentially toxic effects of substances on cultured cells. *In vitro* cytotoxicity and cell viability assays offer several key advantages, particularly when compared to *in vivo* tests. Their rapid execution, lower cost, and ease of automation make them popular choices in drug discovery, toxicology testing, and other biomedical research fields. Moreover, using human cells in these assays can provide more relevant data for human health applications, potentially reducing the need for animal models [5, 6]. By examining how substances interact with cells outside of a living organism, researchers can predict their behavior in biological systems, providing early insights into their safety or potential risks. A key part of this testing is measuring cell viability, which indicates the number of healthy and functioning cells after exposure to a test substance in comparison with an untreated control. Higher cell viability means lower toxicity, while lower viability suggests greater toxicity. Cytotoxicity tests are essential for identifying potentially harmful effects of new compounds, ensuring that only safe candidates proceed to further development.

The accuracy of cytotoxicity testing is paramount, as false negatives can lead to the development of unsafe products, while false positives may discard potentially valuable compounds. Ensuring reliability and reproducibility in these tests is essential for maintaining the integrity of the research process [7, 8]. The ability to measure the number of viable cells represents an important tool with applications in toxicological safety testing, oncological research, industrial microbiology studies, bioprocess monitoring and drug discovery. Recently, increasing evidence has shown some discrepancies between the different methods which has led to either an underestimate or an overestimate of cytotoxicity leading to unreliable toxicity profiles [9].

The choice of assay depends on the specific context of the study, such as the type of cells used, the nature of the substance being tested, and the required sensitivity and specificity. Often, multiple assays are used in combination to provide a more comprehensive understanding of cytotoxicity. With the continuous development of cytotoxicity tests, methods, such as detection of cell damage by morphological changes, determination of cell damage, and measuring cell growth and metabolic properties, have appeared and have gradually been developed from qualitative evaluation to quantitative [8].

Numerous researchers and authors have examined and outlined widely used cell culture assays for studying cytotoxicity. They have categorized the various benefits, drawbacks, and fundamental principles of these methods to promote the standardization and dissemination of comprehensive knowledge, helping researchers make informed decisions when selecting the most suitable approach [10–13].

ISO 10993-5 is a standard for assessing the cytotoxicity of medical devices and materials. However, the standard ISO 10993-5 gives the researcher the great freedom to choose the conditions of the test. Excessive flexibility can lead to a lack of consistency across experiments. This makes it difficult to compare results between different studies, leading to issues with reproducibility and validation of findings. Replicability is a cornerstone of scientific research, ensuring that results are reliable and not just a product of specific, unrepeatable conditions [14]. Standardizing cell culture conditions, including seeding density, media composition, and incubation time, can minimize variability and improve the consistency of results. Regular monitoring of cell health, morphology, and growth rates can help detect any deviations that might impact the outcomes of cytotoxicity assays [14].

A lack of standardization in cytotoxicity testing can lead to several negative consequences, affecting the reliability, reproducibility, and broader application of the results. Different labs may use varying methods, cell lines, and reagents, leading to inconsistent results even when testing the same compound. These inconsistencies can create uncertainty and make it difficult to compare studies across different research groups. Reproducibility is a cornerstone of scientific research. When testing protocols differ between studies, it becomes challenging to replicate findings accurately. This can lead to skepticism about the validity of the data and hinder scientific progress. For drug development and other biotechnological applications, regulatory bodies like the FDA or EMA require reliable and consistent data to evaluate the safety and efficacy of new compounds. Non-standardized tests may not meet regulatory guidelines,

DOI: http://dx.doi.org/10.5772/intechopen.1008312

delaying or complicating the approval process. Inconsistent methods can lead to repeated experiments and wasted resources, including time, money, and materials.

In scientific research, pitfalls are challenges or issues that can hinder progress, lead to inaccurate results, or create inefficiencies. The absence of standardized methods in cytotoxicity assays is one such pitfall, as it can result in unreliable data, poor reproducibility, and inconsistencies that affect both research quality and real-world applications, such as drug development and safety assessments. Addressing pitfalls through standardization efforts would help ensure more reliable, comparable, and translatable results across studies and industries. This chapter addresses common pitfalls in cytotoxicity testing and suggests potential approaches that can help in avoiding them.

2. Potential pitfalls in cytotoxicity testing

Potential pitfalls in cytotoxicity testing can be placed into three identifiable categories, namely: (1) technical challenges, (2) biological factors, and (3) Interpretation of results.

2.1 Technical challenges

2.1.1 Cell culture assays

A study conducted to investigate the proliferative effect of green tea polyphenol showed results obtained from MTT and MTS are different compared to the results obtained from direct measures of ATP and DNA using luminescent cell viability assay kit and cell proliferation assay kit, respectively [15]. The difference is due to the presence of polyphenols that may interfere with the formation of formazan and may change the succinate dehydrogenase activity [15]. Different assays have varying levels of sensitivity and specificity, which can lead to inconsistent results. For example, some assays might detect only late-stage cytotoxicity, missing early signs of cell stress. It's crucial to choose an assay that aligns with the specific objectives of the study and to be aware of its limitations.

2.1.2 Cell line selection

The choice of cell line can significantly influence the outcomes of cytotoxicity testing because different cell lines may respond differently to the same compound due to variations in metabolism, receptor expression, and genetic background [16]. Different cell lines exhibit varying metabolic capacities and enzyme expressions, which can influence how they process or neutralize substances. These differences can affect the cytotoxicity observed. Some cell lines may more effectively convert a pro-drug into its active form, resulting in distinct cytotoxic effects. Relying on a single cell line for cytotoxicity testing may not provide a complete understanding of a substance's overall impact. Various cell lines represent different tissue types and physiological conditions. For example, cancer cell lines like HeLa (cervical cancer) or MCF-7 (breast cancer) may respond differently to drugs compared to normal cell lines like fibroblasts or epithelial cells [17]. The unique genetic profiles, including variations in gene expression, mutations, and signaling pathways can affect how cells respond to cytotoxic agents. For instance, a drug that targets a specific mutation or pathway may be effective in one cell line but not in another that lacks that mutation or pathway [18].

2.1.3 Reagent stability and handling

The stability of reagents, such as dyes, antibodies, and culture media, can affect assay results. Improper storage, repeated freeze–thaw cycles, or contamination can introduce variability. Regular validation of reagent quality and adherence to proper storage and handling protocols are essential to minimize these issues. Dyes used in assays, such as those for viability or proliferation, can degrade over time or with improper storage. For example, a dye like MTT can lose its effectiveness if it is not stored properly [13]. Degradation can lead to inaccurate measurements of cell viability or metabolic activity. Antibodies used in assays, such as ELISA or immunofluorescence, can lose their specificity or affinity if not stored according to manufacturer guidelines. Exposure to incorrect temperatures or repeated freeze–thaw cycles can reduce their effectiveness, leading to false negatives or positives in detection. The stability of culture media is essential for maintaining cell health and experimental consistency. Media components can degrade over time or through improper handling. For instance, the stability of antibiotics, growth factors, and nutrients can affect cell growth and response to treatments, impacting assay outcomes.

Contaminants like bacteria, fungi, or endotoxins can affect reagent performance and introduce variability in assays [19]. Contaminated reagents can lead to inconsistent results or affect cell behavior, skewing the interpretation of cytotoxicity or other tests. Reagents often have specific storage requirements, such as temperature ranges or protection from light. Deviating from these conditions can cause chemical degradation or loss of activity. For instance, some reagents need to be stored at −20°C or lower to prevent degradation. Repeated freeze-thaw cycles can degrade reagents, particularly those that are sensitive to temperature changes, like enzymes or antibodies. It's best to aliquot reagents into smaller portions to avoid repeated freeze-thaw cycles and minimize degradation.

Poor handling of cytotoxicity reagents (e.g., MTT, WST, or CCK-8) can affect their performance. For example, light-sensitive reagents might degrade if exposed to light, or improperly stored reagents can lose potency. In multi-well plates, the edge wells are more prone to evaporation, which can lead to higher concentration of compounds, nutrients, or reduced volume, causing artifacts in the results.

Test material added to the culture medium may adsorb medium components and interfere with nutrient absorption by cells. In a cytotoxicity study by Horie et al. [20], the influence of the adsorption capacity of metal oxide nanoparticles toward medium components was evaluated. The study showed that TiO2 and CeO2 nanoparticles adsorb proteins and Ca ions from the medium.

2.1.4 Concentration and exposure time

Inappropriate concentrations or exposure times can lead to misleading results. High concentrations may cause non-specific cytotoxicity, where the observed effect is due to general cell stress rather than a specific interaction, while too low concentrations might not reveal potential toxic effects. In addition, an excessively high concentration of a cytotoxic agent might kill cells too quickly, making it difficult to measure the true IC_{50} value, while a too-low concentration might not show any effect at all.

Exposure time is critical for assessing the kinetics of drug action or toxicity [11]. Too short an exposure might not allow enough time for the drug to exert its effects, while too long an exposure might lead to secondary effects or cellular adaptation or resistance, altering the response compared to shorter exposures. This can impact the interpretation of the effectiveness or safety of a compound. The timing of the assay endpoint is critical. Cytotoxic effects can vary over time, and an inappropriate endpoint can either miss early toxic effects or fail to capture delayed toxicity. For instance, an early time point might miss cell death that occurs later, while a late time point could overlook reversible effects or adaptive responses.

2.2 Biological factors

2.2.1 Cell density and culture conditions

The density of cells in the culture can impact the results of cytotoxicity assays. At higher cell densities, there may be increased competition for nutrients and oxygen, which can lead to changes in cell metabolism and behavior. This can affect the cell's response to cytotoxic agents and the overall assay results. High cell densities can lead to more significant cell-cell interactions, which might influence how cells respond to treatments. Cells can adhere to each other through various adhesion molecules, such as cadherins, integrins, and selectins. These interactions can influence cell morphology, growth patterns, and responses to treatments [21]. Cells can secrete signaling molecules (such as cytokines, growth factors, or hormones) that act on nearby cells. This type of signaling can influence how cells respond to treatments and how they interact with each other in a culture. When cells reach a high density, they often experience contact inhibition, where cell growth and division are suppressed due to physical contact with neighboring cells. This can impact how cells respond to cytotoxic agents and affect the interpretation of cell proliferation or viability assays. In assays involving immune cells, interactions between immune cells and target cells can affect outcomes. For example, interactions between cytotoxic T cells and cancer cells can influence the effectiveness of immunotherapy or cytotoxic agents [22]. The sensitivity and accuracy of certain assays can be affected by cell density. For example, in assays measuring cell proliferation or viability, very high or very low cell densities can lead to inaccurate readings due to differences in background signal or cell coverage. At high cell densities, the diffusion of reagents (such as dyes or drugs) through the culture medium can be limited, which can impact the effectiveness and accuracy of the assay. For example, a drug might not diffuse effectively to all cells in a densely populated culture. High cell densities can increase the background signal in assays, such as those involving absorbance or fluorescence, which might mask or interfere with the detection of specific effects.

Inaccurate or inconsistent seeding of cells across wells can result in variability in cell density, leading to unreliable data. Many cytotoxic agents act differently depending on the density of cells in culture. For instance, densely packed cells can experience different nutrient access, waste accumulation, and drug exposure than sparsely seeded cells, potentially leading to cell-cell interactions. In high-density cultures, cells communicate through direct contact and secreted signaling molecules (like growth factors or cytokines), which may alter their response to drugs or treatments. High-density cultures may have lower metabolic activity per cell due to limited nutrients or oxygen, affecting the results of assays that depend on measuring metabolic activity (like MTT or XTT assays). The ability of cytotoxic agents to penetrate dense clusters of cells may vary, which can lead to underestimation of a drug's true potency in densely seeded wells. Might show exaggerated toxicity because fewer cells are exposed to the same amount of drug or stress, amplifying the observed effect. High-density wells may show reduced toxicity because the larger cell population buffers the drug's effect or because the assay's readout becomes saturated.

2.2.2 Media composition

The availability of nutrients (e.g., glucose, amino acids, and vitamins) in the culture media affects cell growth, metabolism, and response to treatments. Inadequate nutrients can lead to poor cell health and alter experimental outcomes. The type of cultivation medium is usually dictated by the cell type used, as recommended by the cell depositor. There is a vast number of cultivation media that differ in the constitution and concentration of the components [23]. The variation in the composition of medium can have a pronounced influence on the cytotoxicity results. Besides, many authors do not specify the medium, for example, some claim only "Dulbecco's Modified Eagle Medium (DMEM)" without further specification of glucose concentration or additional buffer content.

Another imprecisely defined but critical factor that could lead to significant inconsistencies is the concentration of fetal bovine serum (FBS) in the medium. FBS contains growth factors, hormones, and nutrients essential for cell growth. Changes in FBS concentration can alter cell proliferation rates, potentially leading to discrepancies in assay results related to cell viability, proliferation, or metabolic activity. FBS proteins can bind to drugs, dyes, or other assay reagents, affecting their bioavailability and efficacy. Changes in FBS concentration can alter the extent of binding, potentially skewing assay results. The concentration of serum proteins, such as albumin or globulins, varies with FBS concentration. These proteins can affect cell adhesion, signaling, and response to treatments, leading to variability in assay outcomes [16].

2.2.3 Acidity/alkalinity

The pH of the culture media affects cellular processes, including enzyme activity, nutrient uptake, and overall cell health. Deviations from the optimal pH range can lead to altered cell behavior and affect assay outcomes. Media often contain buffering agents (e.g., HEPES and bicarbonate) to maintain pH stability. Insufficient buffering can result in pH drift, particularly during prolonged culture periods.

2.2.4 Oxygen/carbon dioxide requirements

Cells require oxygen for aerobic metabolism, and oxygen levels in culture can impact cell growth and function. Low oxygen levels (hypoxia) can simulate tumor microenvironments and affect cell responses, whereas normoxic conditions are typically used for standard cell culture [24]. Hypoxia can influence gene expression and cellular responses, impacting experimental results. Most cell cultures are maintained in a 5% CO_2 environment to regulate pH through bicarbonate buffering. Most cell culture media contain bicarbonate (HCO_3^-) as a buffering agent. The CO_2 in the incubator helps maintain the pH of the culture medium by interacting with bicarbonate to form carbonic acid (H_2CO_3). This buffering system keeps the pH of the media stable, typically around 7.2 to 7.4, which is optimal for most mammalian cells. Without a controlled CO_2 environment, the pH of the medium would drift due to the production of metabolic acids by the cells, leading to potential cell stress or death. The 5% CO_2 level helps maintain the pH within the desired range. CO_2 is a byproduct of cellular respiration and metabolism. Maintaining an appropriate CO_2 level in the incubator ensures that the cell culture environment reflects the metabolic conditions that cells would encounter *in vivo*. A 5% CO_2 environment creates conditions that closely mimic the physiological conditions of the human body, supporting optimal cell growth and function are recommended [25].

2.2.5 Variability due to cell cycle stages

Cells in different stages of the cell cycle may respond differently to toxic agents. For example, cells in the S phase (DNA synthesis) might be more susceptible to certain chemotherapeutics. Administering cytotoxic agents at times when target cells are in a specific cell cycle phase can enhance therapeutic outcomes. For instance, scheduling treatments to coincide with phases where cells are more vulnerable can improve drug efficacy and reduce resistance [26].

2.2.6 Interpretation of results

Background noise from non-specific binding, autofluorescence, or chemical interference can complicate the interpretation of results. This is particularly problematic in assays relying on fluorescence or colorimetric readouts. For example, compounds with inherent color or fluorescence can interfere with colorimetric or fluorescent assays. Certain compounds may interfere with the reagents used in cytotoxicity assays. For example, some drugs might reduce the tetrazolium salt in the MTT assay without requiring cellular metabolism, leading to false-positive results. It's important to include proper controls and to consider potential sources of interference when designing experiments and analyzing data. Relying on the results of a single assay without cross-validation can lead to erroneous conclusions. Different assays might yield conflicting results due to their varying mechanisms of action. Confirming findings with multiple assays or using orthogonal approaches can provide a more robust assessment of cytotoxicity.

2.2.7 Defining the threshold for toxicity

Defining an appropriate threshold for what constitutes "toxic" can be subjective. For example, slight reductions in viability might not be considered toxic in some settings but could be significant in others. The threshold for toxicity refers to the point at which a compound or treatment begins to cause a harmful effect on cells in a cytotoxicity assay. Defining and interpreting this threshold is critical in toxicological research, drug discovery, and safety testing. The toxicity threshold is the concentration or dose of a compound at which there is a measurable decrease in cell viability or a significant toxic effect. Below this threshold, the compound is generally considered non-toxic or safe, while above this level, toxic effects become evident.

3. Strategies to avoid pitfalls

Researchers should carefully select assays that are appropriate for their specific research goals. Assay validation, including testing for linearity, specificity, and reproducibility, is crucial before applying the assay to experimental samples. Pilot studies can help optimize assay conditions and ensure that the selected method will yield reliable results. Positive and negative controls are essential for validating the performance of cytotoxicity assays. They help to distinguish true cytotoxic effects from experimental artifacts, including replicates (biological and technical), which is critical for ensuring the reproducibility and reliability of the data.

3.1 Cell culture selection

Cell lines that mimic the characteristics of the target tissue or disease provide a more biologically relevant environment for studying cellular processes, drug responses, or disease mechanisms [27]. Results obtained from such cell lines are more likely to translate to *in vivo* models or clinical settings, increasing the predictive value of the research. Using a cell line that accurately represents the target tissue can minimize experimental variability and improve the consistency of results.

Ensure the cell line is derived from the same tissue type as the target tissue. If studying a disease, choose a cell line that exhibits genetic or phenotypic characteristics similar to the disease state. Consider the genetic profile of the cell line to ensure it maintains the essential features of the target tissue or disease. Look for well-characterized cell lines with published data on their properties and behavior.

Choose a well-characterized and widely accepted cell line for cytotoxicity testing. Use cells within a narrow passage range (e.g., between 5th and 20th passage) to avoid genetic drift and changes in cellular behavior that occur with prolonged culture [28]. Regularly authenticate cell lines to confirm their identity and purity, ensuring that they have not been contaminated or cross-contaminated with other cell lines.

Researchers must carefully select cell lines that are relevant to the target tissue or disease condition. Using multiple cell lines can help validate findings and get a broader view of cytotoxic effects. Selecting a cell line that closely resembles the target tissue or disease model can make the results more relevant to the intended application.

3.2 Cell culture conditions

Maintain a consistent incubation temperature, typically at 37°C, as cells are sensitive to temperature changes, which can affect their metabolic activity and response to toxicants [29]. Standardization of the CO_2 concentration (usually 5%) in the incubator to maintain the correct pH in the culture medium, as fluctuations can affect cell viability is required. Confirmation of proper humidity levels in the incubator to prevent evaporation of the culture medium, which could concentrate the media components and alter the cells' environment. Maintenance and consistent timing for all steps in the protocol, such as incubation periods, media changes, and time points for measuring cytotoxicity, should be adhered to. Variations in timing can lead to inconsistent results. Reduce the number of times cells are handled or exposed to different environments, as this can stress cells and introduce variability. Handle all samples similarly to ensure uniform exposure to test conditions.

3.3 Culture medium and reagents

Use the same type and batch of culture medium and supplements (e.g., FBS and antibiotics) throughout the experiment. Commonly, FBS concentrations typically range from 5 to 20%, depending on the cell line [16]. Changes in media composition can lead to variations in cell behavior. Where possible, use reagents from the same lot or batch. If changing batches is unavoidable, pre-test the new batch to ensure it produces consistent results with previous ones. Store all media and reagents under appropriate conditions (e.g., refrigeration for serum and room temperature for some buffers) to maintain their stability and effectiveness.

Adherent cell lines require specific media conditions to support their attachment, growth, and proliferation on a surface. Dulbecco's Modified Eagle Medium (DMEM) is a widely used medium for adherent cells and is available in various formulations (e.g., with high or low glucose). It is suitable for a broad range of cell types and supports cell attachment and growth. Eagle's Minimum Essential Medium (MEM): another foundational medium used for adherent cells, with variations that include additional nutrients or vitamins to support specific cell lines, RPMI-1640 is often used for adherent cells, particularly lymphoid and cancer cell lines. It contains higher concentrations of amino acids and vitamins compared to DMEM. To prevent contamination, media may include antibiotics like penicillin and streptomycin or antimycotics like amphotericin B. However, overuse of antibiotics can affect cell behavior and should be minimized. Media for suspended cells, also known as suspension cells, are designed to support cell growth and proliferation in a floating environment rather than adhering to the surface of a culture vessel.

3.4 Seeding density and plate layout

Standardize the number of cells seeded per well. Inconsistent seeding densities can lead to variability in cell confluency and affect the cells' response to toxicants. Ensure even distribution of cells in each well to prevent variations in cell density across the plate. Randomize the placement of samples and controls across the well plate to minimize edge effects or any systematic errors associated with plate positioning [30]. A hemocytometer or an automated cell counter may be used to determine the concentration of cell suspension. This involves taking a small aliquot of your cell suspension, staining it (if necessary), and counting the cells in a defined volume [31]. Regularly monitor the growth of cells in different wells to ensure that they are growing uniformly. Any variations in cell density or behavior might indicate issues with seeding or environmental conditions. Documentation is required for seeding density, volumes used, and any observations about cell behavior or growth including details on the medium used, any supplements added, and the duration of incubation.

3.5 Compound solubility and stability

Insoluble compounds can precipitate in the culture medium, leading to uneven exposure of cells to the compound. This can result in inconsistent cytotoxicity across wells and reduce the accuracy of dose-response data. Techniques such as sonication, the use of solvents, like DMSO, or the addition of surfactants might help, but these approaches can introduce additional variables [32]. Some compounds are unstable and may degrade into other products during the assay. These degradation products might have different cytotoxic profiles than the parent compound, leading to misleading results. Therefore, it is important to confirm the stability of the compound in the culture conditions used and consider potential metabolites that might form. The solvents used to dissolve poorly water-soluble compounds, such as DMSO or ethanol, can themselves be cytotoxic at higher concentrations [33]. It is essential to include vehicle controls to differentiate between the effects of the solvent and the test compound. Even low concentrations of vehicles can have subtle effects on cell physiology that might influence cytotoxicity.

4. Data analysis and interpretation

4.1 Data analysis

Researchers should be cautious when interpreting cytotoxicity data, particularly when dealing with borderline effects. When interpreting cytotoxicity data, particularly in the context of biomaterial testing, researchers must navigate several complexities to ensure that their conclusions are both statistically valid and biologically meaningful. Statistical analysis is essential to determine the significance of observed effects.

Statistical significance determines whether the differences observed between experimental groups (e.g., cells exposed to biomaterial extracts) and control groups are likely to be real or due to random chance. Without statistical analysis, one cannot confidently claim that an observed effect is due to the biomaterial being tested [34]. Commonly used tests include t-tests, which are useful for comparing the means between two groups (e.g., treated vs. untreated cells). ANOVA (Analysis of Variance) is commonly applied when comparing more than two groups or conditions. It helps determine if there are any statistically significant differences among group means. Post-hoc tests are often used after ANOVA to identify specifically which groups differ from each other. A p-value <0.05 is commonly used as a threshold for statistical significance, but this is somewhat arbitrary, and the context of the data should be considered. A statistically significant result means that the observed effect is unlikely to have occurred by chance alone, but it does not confirm that the effect is biologically significant [34].

4.2 Interpretation

IC_{50} (half-maximal inhibitory concentration) and percentage growth inhibition are related concepts in the context of cytotoxicity and drug efficacy studies, but they provide different types of information. Percentage growth inhibition gives detailed insights into how a substance affects cells across different concentrations, while IC50 provides a convenient summary of its overall potency.

4.2.1 Percentage growth inhibition

Percentage growth inhibition is a measure of how much a substance (e.g., drug and biomaterial) inhibits the growth of cells compared to a control group. It is usually calculated at specific concentrations of the test substance [35]. Interpretation: 0% Inhibition: Indicates no effect; the cells are growing as well as in the untreated control. One hundred percent inhibition: Indicates complete inhibition of cell growth; the treated cells have no detectable viability. This metric can be used to express the extent of cytotoxicity or the effect of a drug at specific concentrations, allowing for comparison across different doses.

4.2.2 IC_{50}

IC_{50} is the concentration of a substance that is required to inhibit cell growth or viability by 50% relative to a control [36]. It is a specific value that represents the potency of a substance in terms of its ability to inhibit biological or biochemical function. IC_{50} is determined by plotting the percentage growth inhibition against the logarithm of the concentrations of the test substance and fitting a dose-response curve (often a sigmoidal curve). The IC_{50} is the point on this curve where the inhibition is 50%. Low IC_{50} value: Indicates high potency; a smaller concentration of the substance is needed to inhibit growth by 50%. High IC_{50} Value: Indicates lower potency; a higher concentration is needed to achieve the same level of inhibition. IC_{50} is a key parameter in pharmacology, toxicology, and material science, often used to compare the potency of different substances. The IC_{50} value is essentially derived from a dose-response curve that plots percentage growth inhibition against various concentrations of a substance [37]. Thus, percentage growth inhibition at different concentrations is the underlying data used to calculate IC_{50}.

4.2.3 Selectivity index

The Selectivity Index (SI) is a critical parameter in evaluating the potential of a compound, especially in the field of cancer research and drug development [38]. The therapeutic window is the range of doses at which a compound is effective against disease cells (e.g., cancer) while having minimal toxic effects on healthy cells. The SI is a numerical expression of this window. High SI: Indicates a wide therapeutic window, meaning the compound can be administered at a dose that effectively kills cancer cells while sparing normal cells. This is desirable in anticancer therapies, as it suggests that the compound can target the cancer more specifically without causing significant harm to the patient's healthy tissues. Low SI: Suggests a narrow therapeutic window or poor selectivity, where the compound could be toxic to both cancer and normal cells at similar concentrations, potentially leading to harmful side effects. In drug discovery, SI is used to screen and prioritize compounds based on their selectivity. Compounds with higher SIs are more likely to be selected for further development. Hence, to determine the cytotoxic potential of a compound, Selectivity Index (SI) is used by measuring the ratio of 50% of the inhibitory concentration (IC_{50}) of normal cells to the 50% of cell death population in cancer cells (IC_{50}). The greater the SI value, the more selective it is. If the SI value is >2, the compound is considered to have selective cytotoxic activity. However, if the SI value is <2, it is considered able to give general cytotoxicity toward the cells.

5. Potential future techniques to consider in laboratory testing of cytotoxicity

5.1 Organoids and 3D cell cultures

Organoids and 3D cell cultures represent a significant advancement in cytotoxicity testing. These systems create miniature, self-organizing tissues that closely mimic the architecture and function of actual organs. They offer enhanced physiological relevance, improving the predictive power for drug responses and toxicity. Additionally, organoids can model specific diseases more effectively than traditional 2D cultures and facilitate personalized medicine by using patient-derived cells [39, 40]. However, establishing and maintaining these cultures can be technically challenging and may lead to variability between batches.

5.2 High-content screening (HCS)

High-content screening combines automated microscopy with advanced image analysis to assess multiple cellular parameters simultaneously. This technique allows for a comprehensive analysis of various endpoints, such as cell morphology, viability, and apoptosis, all within the same experiment [41]. HCS enables high-throughput screening of large compound libraries and provides rich datasets that can reveal the subtle effects of cytotoxic agents on cellular processes [42]. Nevertheless, it requires a significant investment in equipment and expertise in data analysis.

5.3 CRISPR/Cas9 gene editing

CRISPR/Cas9 gene editing is a powerful tool for investigating the role of specific genes in cytotoxicity and drug resistance. By allowing precise modifications to targeted genes, researchers can explore the functional consequences of these alterations [43]. This technology facilitates the identification of molecular pathways associated with toxicity, making it invaluable for drug development. However, concerns about off-target effects and ethical implications, particularly regarding germline editing, present challenges that need to be addressed.

5.4 Label-free detection

Label-free detection techniques offer an innovative approach to assessing cytotoxicity without the need for fluorescent or radioactive labels. Methods such as electrical impedance and optical biosensors enable real-time monitoring of cellular responses, providing continuous observation of cell behavior [44]. These techniques are non-invasive and can lead to more accurate assessments of cytotoxicity, although they may be less sensitive than traditionally labeled assays and often require specialized instrumentation [45].

5.5 Single-cell analysis techniques

Single-cell analysis techniques, such as single-cell RNA sequencing, allow researchers to examine individual cell responses to cytotoxic agents. This approach reveals variations in drug responses at the single-cell level, which is critical for understanding the complexities of cellular populations [46]. It also provides insights into unique pathways activated during cytotoxic stress, aiding in biomarker discovery. However, the high costs and technical complexity of single-cell technologies can limit their accessibility.

5.6 Omics technologies

Omics Technologies (proteomics, metabolomics, and transcriptomics) provide comprehensive profiles of the entire set of proteins, metabolites, or RNA in cells, revealing global responses to cytotoxic agents [47, 48]. These technologies offer a holistic view of cellular responses, integrating multiple biological layers and identifying key signaling pathways affected by cytotoxicity. Despite their strengths, omics technologies generate large amounts of data, necessitating advanced bioinformatics skills for interpretation and posing challenges related to standardization.

5.7 Microfluidics

Microfluidics leverages tiny volumes of fluids to manipulate experimental conditions precisely. This technique enables high-throughput screening with minimal sample volumes and allows for the fine-tuning of microenvironments, enhancing the study of cytotoxicity [49]. Microfluidic systems also facilitate single-cell analysis by isolating individual cells for detailed examination. However, designing and fabricating these devices can be complex, and issues such as clogging may complicate experimental setups.

5.8 Artificial intelligence (AI)

Artificial Intelligence and Machine Learning are transforming data analysis in cytotoxicity studies by automating the interpretation of complex datasets [50, 51]. These technologies enhance the ability to predict cellular responses to various compounds based on historical data and can integrate diverse sources of information, providing a comprehensive view of cytotoxicity. Nonetheless, the effectiveness of AI models heavily relies on the quality and quantity of input data, and the models can sometimes act as "black boxes," making it difficult to understand the rationale behind their predictions.

6. Conclusion

Accurate *in vitro* cytotoxicity determination is essential for the early identification of toxic agents, the development of safe drugs, and the advancement of biomedical research. However, the reliability of cytotoxicity assays can be compromised by a range of experimental pitfalls. Through this chapter, we have emphasized the importance of careful assay selection, appropriate control implementation, and the need to optimize experimental conditions to ensure reproducibility and validity of results. Key factors such as serum interference, cell density, solvent toxicity, and compound aggregation must be meticulously managed to avoid generating false-positive or false-negative data. By acknowledging and addressing these challenges, researchers can significantly improve the precision of their cytotoxicity assessments. Ultimately, a well-designed cytotoxicity assay contributes to a more accurate evaluation of a compound's safety profile, paving the way for successful translational research and the development of safer therapeutic agents. Adhering to best practices in cytotoxicity testing will also foster consistency across studies and laboratories, enhancing the reliability of *in vitro* methodologies in toxicological assessments.

Acknowledgements

We would like to thank the University of Limpopo.

Conflict of interest

The authors declare no conflict of interest.

Author details

Mashilo Matotoka and Peter Masoko*
University of Limpopo, Polokwane, South Africa

*Address all correspondence to: peter.masoko@ul.ac.za

References

[1] Sukumaran A, Sweety V, Vikas B, et al. Cytotoxicity and cell viability assessment of biomaterials. In: Cytotoxicity—Understanding Cellular Damage and Response. London, UK: IntechOpen; 2023. DOI: 10.5772/intechopen.111822

[2] Li W, Zhou J, Xu Y. Study of the in vitro cytotoxicity testing of medical devices. Biomedical Reports. 2015;**3**:617-620. DOI: 10.3892/br.2015.481

[3] Eder KM, Marzi A, Wågbø AM, et al. Standardization of an in vitro assay matrix to assess cytotoxicity of organic nanocarriers: A pilot interlaboratory comparison. Drug Delivery and Translational Research. 2022;**12**:2187-2206. DOI: 10.1007/s13346-022-01203-9

[4] Di Nunzio M, Valli V, Tomás-Cobos L, et al. Is cytotoxicity a determinant of the different in vitro and in vivo effects of bioactives? BMC Complementary and Alternative Medicine. 2017;**17**:453. DOI: 10.1186/s12906-017-1962-2

[5] Kunzmann A, Andersson B, Thurnherr T, Krug H, Scheynius A, Fadeel B. Toxicology of engineered nanomedical devices: Focus on biocompatibility, biodistribution and biodegradation. Biochimica et Biophysica Acta. 2011;**1810**:361-373. DOI: 10.1016/j.bbagen.2010.04.007

[6] Ukelis U, Kramer P-J, Olejniczak K, Mueller SO. Replacement of in vivo acute oral toxicity studies by in vitro cytotoxicity methods: Opportunities, limits and regulatory status. Regulatory Toxicology and Pharmacology. 2008;**51**:108-118

[7] Niles AL, Moravec RA, Riss TL. In vitro viability and cytotoxicity testing and same-well multi-parametric combinations for high throughput screening. Current Chemical Genomics. 2009;**3**:33-41. DOI: 10.2174/1875397300903010033

[8] Escher BI, Neale PA, Villeneuve DL. The advantages of linear concentration-response curves for in vitro bioassays with environmental samples. Environmental Toxicology and Chemistry. 2018;**37**:2273-2280. DOI: 10.1002/etc.4178

[9] Rajalingam R. The impact of HLA class I-specific killer cell immunoglobulin-like receptors on antibody-dependent natural killer cell-mediated cytotoxicity and organ allograft rejection. Frontiers in Immunology. 2016;**7**:585. DOI: 10.3389/fimmu.2016.00585

[10] Aslantürk ÖS. In Vitro Cytotoxicity and Cell Viability Assays: Principles, Advantages, and Disadvantages. London, UK: InTech Open; 2018. DOI: 10.5772/intechopen.71923

[11] Gutleb AC, Morrison E, Murk AJ. Cytotoxicity assays for mycotoxins produced by fusarium strains: A review. Environmental Toxicology and Chemistry. 2002;**11**:309-320. DOI: 10.1016/s1382-6689(02)00020-0

[12] Brioschi MBC, Coser EM, Coelho AC, Gadelha FR, Miguel DC. Models for cytotoxicity screening of antileishmanial drugs: What has been done so far? International Journal of Antimicrobial Agents. 2022;**60**:106612. DOI: 10.1016/j.ijantimicag.2022.106612

[13] Riss T, Niles A, Moravec R, et al. Cytotoxicity assays: In vitro methods to measure dead cells. 2019 may 1. In: Markossian S, Grossman A, Arkin M,

et al., editors. Assay Guidance Manual [Internet]. Eli Lilly & Company and the National Center for Advancing Translational Sciences: Bethesda (MD); 2004

[14] Shafiee MAM, Asri MAM, Alwi SSS. Review on the cytotoxicity assessment in accordance to the International Organization for Standardization (ISO). Malaysian Journal of Medical Research. 2021;**17**:261-269

[15] Wang P, Henning SM, Heber D. Limitations of MTT and MTS-based assays for measurement of antiproliferative activity of green tea polyphenols. PLoS One. 2010;**5**:e10202. DOI: 10.1371/journal.pone.0010202

[16] Baker M. Reproducibility: Respect your cells! Nature. 2016;**537**:433-435. DOI: 10.1038/537433a

[17] Tran V, Kim R, Maertens M, Hartung T, Maertens A. Similarities and differences in gene expression networks between the breast cancer cell line Michigan cancer foundation-7 and invasive human breast cancer tissues. Frontiers in Artificial Intelligence. 2021;**4**:674370. DOI: 10.3389/frai.2021.674370

[18] Witt BL, Tollefsbol TO. Molecular, cellular, and technical aspects of breast cancer cell lines as a foundational tool in cancer research. Life. 2023;**13**:2311. DOI: 10.3390/life13122311

[19] Weiskirchen S, Schröder SK, Buhl EM, Weiskirchen R. A beginner's guide to cell culture: Practical advice for preventing needless problems. Cells. 2023;**12**:682. DOI: 10.3390/cells12050682

[20] Horie M, Nishio K, Fujita K, Endoh S, Miyauchi A, Saito Y, et al. Protein adsorption of ultrafine metal oxide and its influence on cytotoxicity toward cultured cells. Chemical Research in Toxicology. 2009;**22**:543-553. DOI: 10.1021/tx800289z

[21] Khalili AA, Ahmad MR. A review of cell adhesion studies for biomedical and biological applications. International Journal of Molecular Sciences. 2015;**16**:18149-18184. DOI: 10.3390/ijms160818149

[22] Ahmed H, Mahmud AR, Siddiquee MF, Shahriar A, Biswas P, Shimul MEK, et al. Role of T cells in cancer immunotherapy: Opportunities and challenges. Cancer Pathogensis and Therapy. 2022;**1**:116-126. DOI: 10.1016/j.cpt.2022

[23] Golikov MV, Valuev-Elliston VT, Smirnova OA, Ivanov AV. Physiological media in studies of cell metabolism. Molecular Biology. 2022;**56**(5):629-637. DOI: 10.1134/S0026893322050077

[24] Hulikova A, Vaughan-Jones RD, Swietach P. Dual role of $CO_2/HCO_3(-)$ buffer in the regulation of intracellular pH of three-dimensional tumor growths. The Journal of Biological Chemistry. 2011;**286**:13815-13826. DOI: 10.1074/jbc.M111.219899

[25] Price A, Coecke S. Guidance on good cell culture practice (GCCP). In: Aschner M, Suñol C, Bal-Price A, editors. Cell Culture Techniques. New York, USA: Springer; 2011. pp. 1-25

[26] Granada AE, Jiménez A, Stewart-Ornstein J, Blüthgen N, Reber S, Jambhekar A, et al. The effects of proliferation status and cell cycle phase on the responses of single cells to chemotherapy. Molecular Biology of the Cell. 2020;**31**:845-857. DOI: 10.1091/mbc.E19-09-0515

[27] Skrzydlewski P, Twarużek M, Grajewski J. Cytotoxicity of mycotoxins

and their combinations on different cell lines: A review. Toxins. 2022;**244**. DOI: 10.3390/toxins14040244

[28] Neumann E, Riepl B, Knedla A, Lefèvre S, Tarner IH, Grifka J, et al. Cell culture and passaging alters gene expression pattern and proliferation rate in rheumatoid arthritis synovial fibroblasts. Arthritis Research & Therapy. 2010;**12**:83. DOI: 10.1186/ar3010

[29] Gutierrez C, Somoskovi A, Natarajan K, Bell D. Need for better adherence to optimal incubation temperature for quality laboratory diagnostics and antibiotic resistance monitoring. African Journal of Laboratory Medicine. 2018;**7**(2):789. DOI: 10.4102/ajlm.v7i2.789

[30] Kusena JWT, Shariatzadeh M, Studd AJ, James JR, Thomas RJ, Wilson SL. The importance of cell culture parameter standardization: An assessment of the robustness of the 2102Ep reference cell line. Bioengineered. 2021;**12**:341-357. DOI: 10.1080/21655979.2020.1870074

[31] Piccinini F, Tesei A, Arienti C, Bevilacqua A. Cell counting and viability assessment of 2D and 3D cell cultures: Expected reliability of the Trypan blue assay. Biological Procedures Online. 2017;**19**:8. DOI: 10.1186/s12575-017-0056-3

[32] Selvakumar P, Karthik V, Kumar PS, Asaithambi P, Kavitha S, Sivashanmugam P. Enhancement of ultrasound assisted aqueous extraction of polyphenols from waste fruit peel using dimethyl sulfoxide as surfactant: Assessment of kinetic models. Chemosphere. 2021;**263**:128071. DOI: 10.1016/j.chemosphere.2020.128071

[33] Ilieva Y, Dimitrova L, Zaharieva MM, Kaleva M, Alov P, Tsakovska I, et al. Cytotoxicity and microbicidal activity of commonly used organic solvents: A comparative study and application to a standardized extract from vaccinium macrocarpon. Toxics. 2021;**9**:92. DOI: 10.3390/toxics9050092

[34] Dahiru T. P—Value, a true test of statistical significance? A cautionary note. Annals of Ibadan Postgraduate Medicine. 2008;**6**:21-26. DOI: 10.4314/aipm.v6i1.64038

[35] Larsson P, Engqvist H, Biermann J, Werner Rönnerman E, Forssell-Aronsson E, Kovács A, et al. Optimization of cell viability assays to improve replicability and reproducibility of cancer drug sensitivity screens. Scientific Reports. 2020;**10**:5798. DOI: 10.1038/s41598-020-62848-5

[36] Berrouet C, Dorilas N, Rejniak KA, Tuncer N. Comparison of drug inhibitory effects ([formula: See text]) in monolayer and spheroid cultures. Bulletin of Mathematical Biology. 2020;**82**:68. DOI: 10.1007/s11538-020-00746-7

[37] Garcia-Molina P, Garcia-Molina F, Teruel-Puche JA, Rodriguez-Lopez JN, Garcia-Canovas F, Muñoz-Muñoz JL. The relationship between the IC50 values and the apparent inhibition constant in the study of inhibitors of tyrosinase diphenolase activity helps confirm the mechanism of inhibition. Molecules. 2022;**27**:3141. DOI: 10.3390/molecules27103141

[38] Smolobochkin A, Niyazova D, Gazizov A, Syzdykbayev M, Voloshina A, Amerhanova S, et al. Discovery of Di(het)arylmethane and dibenzoxanthene derivatives as potential anticancer agents. International Journal of Molecular Sciences. 2024;**25**:6724. DOI: 10.3390/ijms25126724

[39] Urzì O, Gasparro R, Costanzo E, De Luca A, Giavaresi G, Fontana S, et al. Three-dimensional cell cultures: The bridge between In vitro and In vivo models. International Journal of Molecular Sciences. 2023;**24**:12046. DOI: 10.3390/ijms241512046

[40] Fang Y, Eglen RM. Three-dimensional cell cultures in drug discovery and development. SLAS Discovery. 2017;**22**:456-472. DOI: 10.1177/1087057117696795

[41] Martin HL, Adams M, Higgins J, Bond J, Morrison EE, Bell SM, et al. High-content, high-throughput screening for the identification of cytotoxic compounds based on cell morphology and cell proliferation markers. PLoS One. 2014;**9**:e88338. DOI: 10.1371/journal.pone.0088338

[42] Mandavilli BS, Aggeler RJ, Chambers KM. Tools to measure cell health and cytotoxicity using high content imaging and analysis. Methods in Molecular Biology. 2018;**1683**:33-46. DOI: 10.1007/978-1-4939-7357-6_3

[43] Li W, Huang C, Chen J. The application of CRISPR /Cas mediated gene editing in synthetic biology: Challenges and optimizations. Frontiers in Bioengineering and Biotechnology. 2022;**10**:890155. DOI: 10.3389/fbioe.2022.890155

[44] Kühn J, Shaffer E, Mena J, Breton B, Parent J, Rappaz B, et al. Label-free cytotoxicity screening assay by digital holographic microscopy. Assay and Drug Development Technologies. 2013;**11**:101-107. DOI: 10.1089/adt.2012.476

[45] Meindl C, Absenger M, Roblegg E, Fröhlich E. Suitability of cell-based label-free detection for cytotoxicity screening of carbon nanotubes. BioMed Research International. 2013;**2013**:564804. DOI: 10.1155/2013/564804

[46] Cham LB, Gunst JD, Schleimann MH, Frattari GS, Rosas-Umbert M, Vibholm LK, et al. Single cell analysis reveals a subset of cytotoxic-like plasmacytoid dendritic cells in people with HIV-1. iScience. 2023;**26**:107628. DOI: 10.1016/j.isci.2023.107628

[47] Gao YN, Yang X, Wang JQ, Liu HM, Zheng N. Multi-omics reveal additive cytotoxicity effects of aflatoxin B1 and aflatoxin M1 toward intestinal NCM460 cells. Toxins (Basel). 2022;**14**:368. DOI: 10.3390/toxins14060368

[48] Cheng D, Deng B, Tong Q, Gao S, Xiao B, Zhu M, et al. Proteomic studies of the mechanism of cytotoxicity, induced by palytoxin on HaCaT cells. Toxins (Basel). 2022;**14**:269. DOI: 10.3390/toxins14040269

[49] Fan XY, Deng ZF, Yan YY, Orel E, Shypko A, Orel V, et al. Application of microfluidic chips in anticancer drug screening. Bosnian Journal of Basic Medical Sciences. 2022;**22**:302-314. DOI: 10.17305/bjbms.2021

[50] Basile AO, Yahi A, Tatonetti NP. Artificial intelligence for drug toxicity and safety. Trends in Pharmacological Sciences. 2019;**40**:624-635. DOI: 10.1016/j.tips.2019.07.005

[51] Russo V, Lallo E, Munnia A, Spedicato M, Messerini L, D'Aurizio R, et al. Artificial intelligence predictive models of response to cytotoxic chemotherapy alone or combined to targeted therapy for metastatic colorectal cancer patients: A systematic review and meta-analysis. Cancers (Basel). 2022;**14**:4012. DOI: 10.3390/cancers14164012

Chapter 4

Exploring the Effects of Seaweed Synthesized Nanoparticles on Human Cancer Cell Lines

Pitchai Palaniappan, Kannaiah Surendirakumar, Manoharan Ravi and Ramar Ramesh

Abstract

Seaweeds can be found in either marine or brackish water and have the potential to be bioactive. Seaweeds are important ecological, biological, and regenerative components of the maritime environment. Because of their high concentration of polysaccharides and phytochemicals, they have sparked a lot of interest in the domains of cosmetics, biomass for fuels, and as a source material for nanoparticle synthesis. Phytochemicals found in seaweeds aid in the conversion of metal ions to nanoparticles, which can easily overcome the tumor micro-environment barrier and cause damage in cancer cells. In addition, nanotechnology-based medicine has a promising therapeutic effect in cancer treatment. Functionalized nanoparticles improve the therapeutic effects of anticancer drugs while also delivering them to the tumor site over time. Metal nanoparticles have sparked a lot of attention in the scientific community for their use in biomedical nanotechnology. Drug-loaded metal nanoparticles were more hazardous to cancer cells than bare anticancer drugs.

Keywords: marine nanotechnology, cytotoxicity, apoptosis, nanoparticles, bioactive compounds, seaweeds, reducing agents

1. Introduction

In the twenty-first century, nanotechnology is widely employed globally. Nanotechnology has benefited several areas, including medical (health) care, biological studies, safety, and nanoelectronics [1]. Macroalgae, known for their many biological roles, are believed to include numerous unexplored bioactive chemical compounds. Seaweeds are the most abundant multicellular marine macroalgae. Seaweeds have a high fiber and protein content [2]. A hydrocolloid layer recognizes a large number of polysaccharides, including structural polysaccharides in cell walls. Agar and alginate for brown algae. Storage polysaccharides such as laminarin are found in seaweeds [3]. Nanoparticles with inherent antibacterial and anticancerous capabilities, such as silver and gold, have recently been employed in medicinal treatment [4–6]. Zinc oxide (ZnO) nanoparticles (NPs) are valuable metal oxides due to their unique chemicals. Commercial utilization for ZnO-NPs include catalysis, solar power cells, biological science, and the beauty sector [7]. Nanoparticle production has negative environmental implications, time-consuming processes, and high costs. Physical and chemical approaches are often associated with undesirable results [6]. Conventional nanoparticle synthesis procedures often result in unstable particles because of their high reactive and surface energy properties. Green nanoparticle synthesis is an eco-friendly and cost-effective solution to alleviate environmental contaminants [7]. "Phyconanotechnology" (PhycoNTs) is an alternate approach for synthesizing nanoparticles. Phyconanotechnology is the process of synthesizing nanomaterials from algae biomass and proteins [8]. There are several advantages to using seaweed to synthesize nanoparticles. Seaweed is a renewable resource that functions as an environmentally friendly (natural) stabilizer and reductive agent, minimizing the necessity of chemicals that are harsh. This technique is ecologically friendly, cost-effective, and scalable, making it suitable for mass production. Seaweed extracts contain bioactive components that enhance the unique properties of produced nanoparticles, rendering them appropriate for use in medicine, agriculture, environmental remediation, etc. (**Figure 1**) [9–11].

Cancer is among the main causes of death on the globe [12]. WHO (World Health Organization) and IARC (International Agency for Research on Cancer) have issued the most recent worldwide cancer burden estimates for around 115 countries. According to IARC projections, the cancer burden is increasing, vulnerable people are particularly susceptible, and there is an urgent need to address cancer disparities globally. In 2022, 20 million new cancer diagnoses occurred, with 9.7 million deaths. More than 35 million additional cancer cases are projected in 2050, a 77% increase over the estimated 20 million in 2022. The fast-increasing worldwide cancer burden reflects both population aging and expansion, exposure to potentially harmful factors, and social and economic progress [13–15]. Current cancer strategies include postoperative treatment and multimodal therapy such as chemotherapy, surgery, and radiotherapy [16]. Chemotherapeutic agents exhibit low efficiency due to the immunosuppressive mechanism of cancer cells, which is the major obstacle in the development of nanodrug strategy. The resistance of tumor cells can overcome the anticancer efficacy of commercial chemotherapeutics [17, 18]. Due to a lack of public understanding, insufficient healthcare facilities, and limited funds, the situation could potentially become worse. Seaweed compounds have recently received attention as an advantageous resource for the synthesis of nanostructures with enhanced anticancer capabilities [9, 19–23].

The present review offers a comprehensive summary of the latest progress in understanding the cytotoxicity, or anticancer properties, of three main categories of marine macroalgae (Seaweeds): green algae (Chlorophyta), brown algae (Phaeophyceae), and red algae (Rhodophyta). These macroalgae have been studied in relation to various types of cancers, including breast, lung, pancreatic, liver, cervical, colorectal, gastric, leukemia, melanoma, etc. Furthermore, this paper also addresses future prospects and constraints in this particular area of study. A cytotoxicity test is a biological evaluation and screening test that employs tissue cells *in vitro* to observe the cellular growth, reproduction, and morphological impacts caused by medical devices [24]. Cytotoxicity is one of the most essential approaches for biological evaluation since it has a number of advantages, including being preferred and necessary. Nanoparticle (NP) cytotoxicity testing is regarded as a vital step toward their

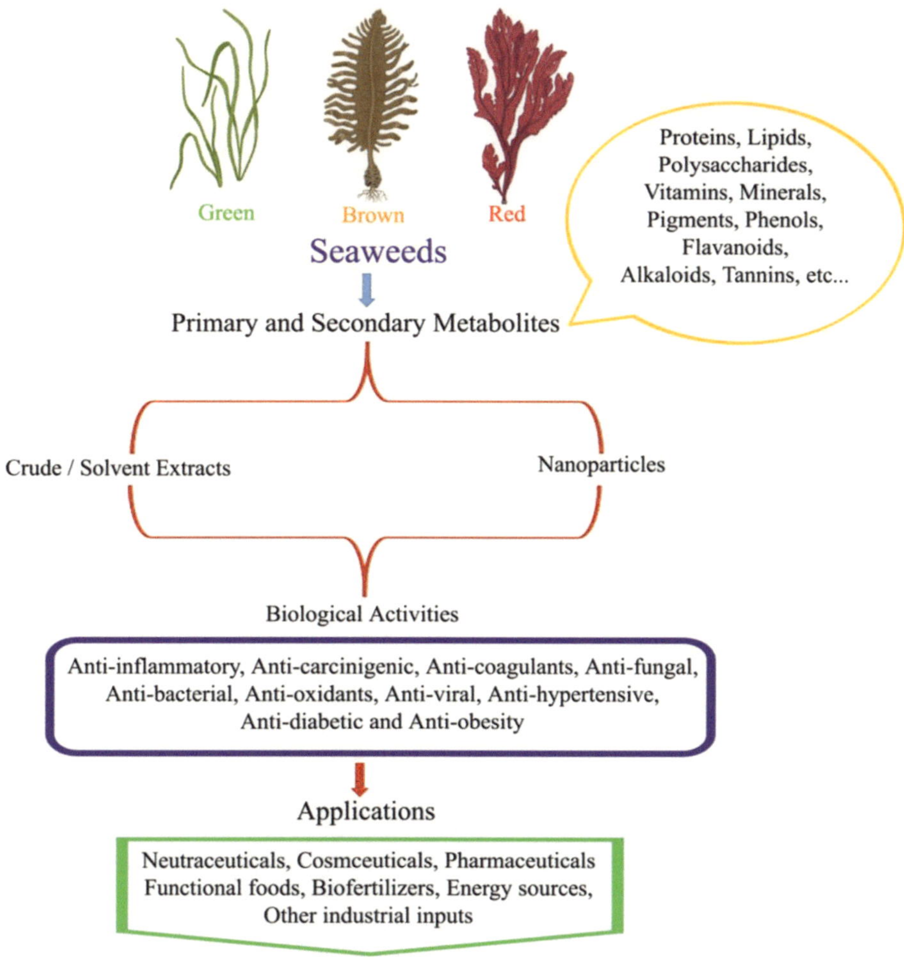

Figure 1.
A schematic overview of seaweed primary and secondary metabolites and their potential applications as bioactive substances in various fields.

effective use in the biomedical industry. However, traditional experimental methods for cytotoxicity measures are frequently costly, time-consuming, and necessitate extensive cell culture training. Generally, seaweeds and their bioactive components have a broad biological application. Because of the extreme environmental circumstances in the marine bionetwork, marine seaweed produces a variety of bioactive chemicals in order to survive.

2. Green synthesis of nanoparticles using green, brown, and red seaweeds

Macroalgae (seaweeds) may synthesize metallic nanoparticles such as silver, gold, platinum, iron oxide, and copper oxide. Seaweeds are an ideal alternative for biogenesis of nanoparticles due to their ability to gather metals and reduce ions. These "bionano factories" produce metallic nanoparticles using both living and dry biomass (**Figure 2**) [25]. Recent research shows that silver can be converted into nanoparticles

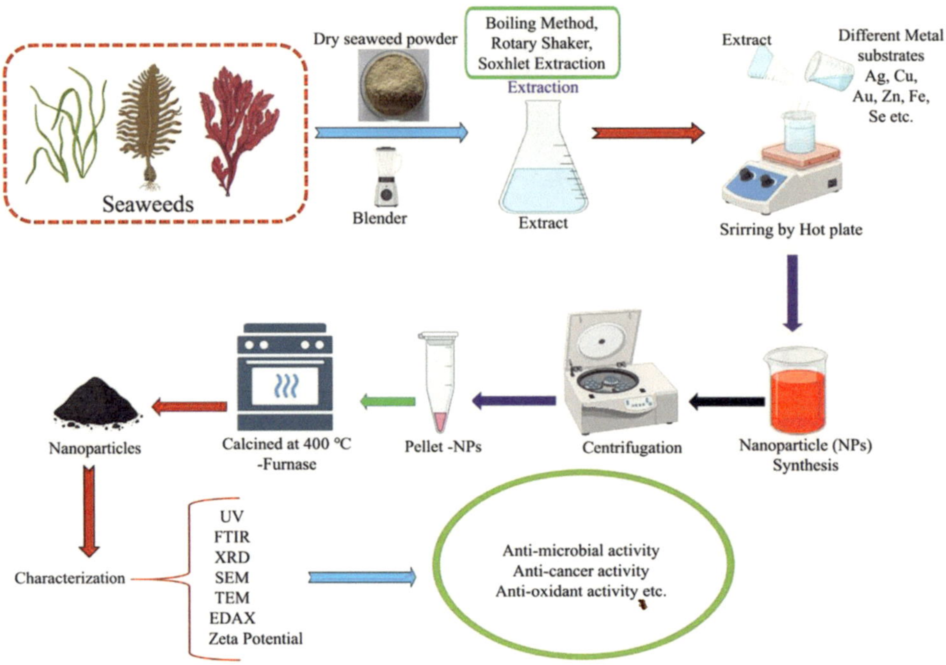

Figure 2.
Biosynthesis of nanoparticles using seaweeds.

by *Cymodocea serrulata*, *Enteromorpha compressa*, *Cystoseira myrica*, *Sargassum polycystum*, *Sargassum vulgare*, *Turbinaria conoides*, *Turbinaria ornata*, *Champia parvula*, etc. [26–31]. Gold nanoparticles were synthesized using *Caulerpa racemosa*, *Codium tomentosum*, *Gracilaria edulis*, *Sargassum wightii*, *Turbinaria conoides*, *Acanthophora spicifera*, *Champia parvula*, *Corallina officinalis*, *Gracilaria verrucosa*, *Hypnea valentiae*, etc. [10, 32–37]. *Caulerpa sertularioides* is utilized for the biosynthesis of zinc nanoparticles [38]. The iron nanoparticles were synthesized by *Sargassum muticum*, *Spatoglossum asperum*, and *Dictyota dicotoma* [39–41]. Magnesium oxide nanoparticles were also synthesized using the aqueous extract of *Sargassum wightii* and *Cystoseira crinita* [42, 43].

3. Mechanism for biosynthesis of nanoparticles utilizing seaweeds

Nanoparticles can be synthesized via numerous methods, including biological, physical, chemical, and hybrid processes. Chemical and physical procedures are extensively utilized for nanoparticle manufacturing; however, their applicability is limited due to the use of toxic materials [5]. All forms of seaweed (green, brown, and red) can absorb heavy metals in higher amounts and change morphology [25]. To reduce toxicity during nanoparticle manufacturing, eco-friendly green technologies are crucial [2]. Physical parameters like pH, temperature, incubation and reaction time, concentration of extract (precursor) affect the formation, development, and stability of nanomaterials and can be altered to control particle morphological qualities (shape and size) and prevent agglomeration [44]. Seaweeds contain phytochemicals that reduce metal ions and stabilize and cap them [5]. **Figure 2** depicts the process of producing nanoparticles using seaweed.

4. Biosynthesis of metal and metal oxide nanoparticles using seaweeds

4.1 Extraction methods

The first stage in nanoparticle synthesis involves extracting algae components with solvents. Solvent extraction was done using boiling, rotational shaking, and Soxhlet extraction [5, 45]. Pugazhendhi et al. [43] found that boiling was the preferred extraction method for synthesizing silver nanoparticles from *Sargassum wightii*. In addition, Silver nanoparticles were synthesized from *Padina pavonica* extract via Soxhlet extraction. *Padina pavonica* dry biomass was crushed and combined with solvent in a Soxhlet extractor for 20 hours [46]. A recent study employed a rotary shaker to produce copper nanoparticles from the algae *Bifurcaria bifurcate*. A recent study employed a rotary shaker to produce copper nanoparticles from the algae *B. bifurcate* [47].

4.2 Solvents utilized

Reaction mixtures typically contain 75% solvent. Metal ions must be reduced, transformed, and nucleated in the liquid phase during nanoparticle production. Solvents remove chemicals from algae, reducing their size. The solvents employed in the technique will influence the size, form, and stability of the nanoparticles (NPs). Water is widely used for brown seaweed-mediated nanoparticle production. Aqueous extract can be used to produce silver (Ag), gold (Au), copper oxide (CuO), and zinc oxide (ZnO) NPs in an environmentally acceptable manner, according to studies. Metal and metal oxide nanoparticles were synthesized using alcohols such as methanol and ethanol, along with other solvents. According to a recent study, *Padina pavonica* ethanol extract produced silver nanoparticles that had different shapes and sizes, including spheres, pyramids, hexagons, and rods, with sizes ranging from 1 to 49.5 nm. In contrast, *Padina pavonica* with chloroform extract manufactured spherical silver nanoparticles with an average size of 0.8 nm [46]. The study found that solvents play a significant role in the creation of nanoparticles, with varying morphologies depending on the solvent employed for extraction.

4.3 Phytochemicals

Seaweed extract contains phytochemicals that effectively reduce metal to nanoparticles. Seaweed extracts contain phenols, flavonoids, alkaloids, terpenes, and polyphenolic derivatives like ascorbic acid and citric acid, which are effective reducing agents in NPs formation [36]. The phytochemical content in the extract varies between algae species, influencing nanoparticle formation, shape, size, and activity [48, 49]. *Gracilaria edulis* extract contains phenolic chemicals that reduce and synthesize silver nanoparticles [33]. Laminarin, a polysaccharide derived from *Turbinaria ornata*, was used to produce silver nanoparticles [31]. *Sargassum muticum*'s crude fucoidan can convert gold into nanoparticles [47]. **Figure 2** shows the phytochemicals and extracts used to produce seaweed nanoparticles.

5. Factors affecting the synthesis of NPs

Factors like pH, temperature, reaction time, plant extract concentration, and metal ion concentration afect the seaweed-based biosynthesis of nanoparticles [27]. pH has an important role in the production of NPs. The pH levels of the reaction solution between seaweed extract and metal ions affect the production, shape, and stability of NPs. The formation of nucleation centers accelerates as the reaction mixture's pH rises. The creation of nucleation sites leads to increased metal transition to nanoparticles. Chandran et al. [39] discovered seaweed -*Dictyota dichotoma* produced iron (Fe) nanoparticles only at pH levels ranging from 7 to 10. In contrast, Namvar et al. [40] generated iron oxide nanoparticles using *Sargassum muticum* under normal pH conditions. Temperature is an important aspect to consider while synthesizing nanoparticles. Recent studies show that seaweed-assisted NPs could be generated at various temperatures. According to studies, nanoparticles develop more slowly at normal temperature than at high temperatures [29]. Ag-NPs from *Sargassum polycystum* and *S. wightii* formed after 24–48 hours at room temperature [29, 48]. Au-NPs were synthesized from *Scytosiphon lomentaria* under five different temperature conditions, with the greatest yield at 100°C [50]. The synthesis of seaweed NPs relies heavily on reaction time. Deepak et al. [48] found that Ag-NPs developed after 24 hours of room temperature incubation in *Sargassum wightii*. In contrast, *Sargassum polycystum* found that silver nanoparticles can be formed over 24–48 hours [29]. Moreover, concentration of seaweed extract also affects the conversion of metal ions into NPs. A recent study found that Au-NPs could be biosynthesized with 0.5 mL of *Lobophora variegate* extract. In contrast, *Dictyota dicotoma* algae extract (10 mL) is used to manufacture FeO-NPs [39]. In addition, Salt content, that is, metal ions is the most crucial factor in nanoparticle production. Au-NPs were synthesized using *Sargassum longifolium* and *Turbina conoides* algae extracts at 20 and 10 mg/L of gold chloride solutions [51].

6. Characterization of seaweed synthesized NPs

Nanoparticles are identified by their shape, size, and dispersion [41]. UV-visible spectroscopy was mostly used for the first confirmation of produced nanoparticles. The nanoparticles were analyzed using XRD to assess their crystalline structure and size. X-rays penetrate nanoparticles and confirm their structure by comparing the observed diffraction pattern to the standard (JCPDS number) [46]. FTIR was utilized to evaluate the available functional groups that contribute to nanoparticle formation. The extract and synthesized NPs were assessed independently at 4000 to 400 cm^{-1}. FTIR data identifies functional chemical complexes in seaweed extract and confirms their role in biosynthesis for NPs [4]. FE-SEM and EDX were utilized to determine the elemental content and percentage of generated seaweed nanoparticles, as well as their surface shape [10].

7. Anticancer activity of green synthesized nanoparticles

Nanoparticles are therapeutic compounds used to diagnose and cure cancer. Nanoparticles are more hazardous to cancer cells than bulk materials. Nanoparticles have been shown to block cancer cell progression through several signaling cascades,

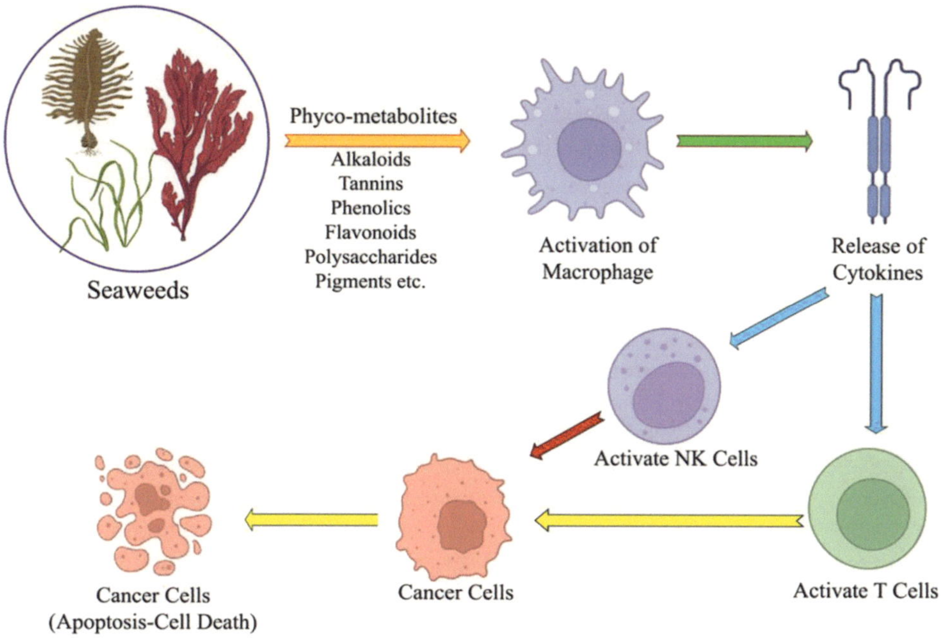

Figure 3.
Cytotoxicity and apoptosis processes of seaweed nanoparticles.

which are crucial for cancer development and pathogenesis (**Figure 3**). Nanoparticles have no fatal effect on normal cells [34, 52].

7.1 Green seaweeds

Palaniappan et al. [34] synthesized gold nanoparticles (Au-NPs) using "sea grapes," that is, *Caulerpa racemosa* extract, in a simple, quick, and ecologically benign biogenic approach. The Au-NPs demonstrated cytotoxicity against H460 (lung cancer cells) with an IC_{50} value of 25 μg/mL. Au-NPs produced from *C. racemosa* extract activate apoptosis through many routes, including extrinsic, intrinsic, and mitochondrial. Similarly, Ragunath et al. [53] generated Ag-NPs from *Caulerpa racemosa* and found dose-dependent cytotoxicity against MCF-7 (breast cancer cells), with an IC_{50} value of 38 μg/mL. Agena et al. [9] found that *Caulerpa sertularioides* (CSE) phytochemicals had a substantial impact on cell survival, apoptosis, cell cycle, and tumor invasion in the SKLU-1 (lung adenocarcinoma cell line), with an IC_{50} value of 80.28 μg/mL. Further, CSE reduced mitochondrial membrane potential, triggered apoptosis via extrinsic and intrinsic routes, elevated caspases-3 and -7, and dramatically reduced tumor invasion in SKLU-1 and induces biochemical and morphological alterations in the plasma membrane, as well as cell cycle arrest in the S, G2/M stages, etc. Nova et al. [52] reported the phytochemical components, antioxidant (DPPH), and anticancer capabilities of MCF-7 and MDA-MB-231 (breast cancer cell lines) of *Chaetomorpha* sp. Quach et al. [54] isolated sulfated galacton polysaccharides (SGP) from *Codium geppiorum*. The SGP showed substantial cytotoxic action on HT29, 8505c, and HeLa (colorectal adenocarcinoma, undifferentiated thyroid carcinomas, and cervical cancer cell lines) with IC_{50} values of 51.8, 89.3, and 72.2 μg/mL, respectively. Palaniappan et al. [28] synthesized bioactive Ag-NPs by *Cymodocea serrulata*. Higher temperatures resulted in maximum Ag-NPs compared to room temperature (37°C) and refrigerator conditions (–20°C). *C. serrulata* Ag-NPs exhibit significant cytotoxicity against A549 (human lung cancer) cells. Ramkumar et al. [30] used *Enteromorpha compressa* seaweed extract to produce biocompatible and functionalized Ag-NPs. The produced Ag-NPs exhibited positive cytotoxicity with EAC (Ehlrich Ascites Carcinoma) cells (IC_{50} = 95.3 μg/mL). Mohanta et al. [33] produced Ag-NPs using *Gracilaria edulis* (seaweed) and were nearly spherical in form. The DPPH, hydroxyl radical, ABTS, and nitric oxide radical-scavenging experiments demonstrated that the produced nanoparticles have substantial antioxidant capabilities. The *G. edulis*-mediated Ag-NPs revealed dose-dependent cytotoxicity against MDA-MB-231 (IC_{50} of 344.27 ± 2.56 μg/mL). Similarly, Akter et al. [55] previously demonstrated that Ag-NPs generated from *G. edulis* exhibited valuable cytotoxicity with MDA-MB-231 cells (IC_{50} of 21.2 μg/mL). Husni et al. [56] investigated the cytotoxic activity of *Halimeda tuna* methanol crude extract against A549 cells (IC_{50} = 2771 μg/mL). Thanh et al. [45] used ultrasound to extract *Ulva lactuca* polysaccharides "Ulvan." The ulvan has shown cytotoxic activity against five human cancer cell lines (human hepatocellular carcinoma, breast cancer, cervical cancer, colorectal adenocarcinoma, and undifferentiated thyroid carcinoma). Furthermore, Alshehri and Panneerselvam [57] initially reported the manufacture of graphene oxide (GO) nanoparticles using *Ulva lactuca*. The test results reveal that the apoptotic behavior of graphene derivatives in the MCF-7 cell line increases with sample concentration. This research could provide new light on the antibacterial, antioxidant, and anticancer properties of green-produced graphene-based compounds. Güler et al. [22] found that the ethanol extract of *Ulva rigida* had a considerable cytotoxic effect on human cervical adenocarcinoma (HeLa) cells (IC_{50} = 21 μg/mL) and modest anti-angiogenic activity (0.98 at 50 μM) (**Table 1**).

7.2 Brown seaweeds

Mohamed et al. [27] suggested an environmentally acceptable method of biosynthesizing silver nanoparticles from *Cystoseira myrica*. Silver nanoparticles' cytotoxicity against MCF-7 and HepG2 was tested at varied doses. The maximal percentage of viability against MCF-7 and HepG2 cell lines fell from 94.5 to 19.8 and from 78.5 to 25.8 following time exposure, respectively. Namvar et al. [40] produced iron oxide (Fe_3O_4) nanoparticles using an aqueous extract of the brown seaweed *Sargassum muticum*. Fe_3O_4-NPs showed cytotoxic effects on chemotherapy-resistant ovarian cancer cells – A2780cp (IC_{50} values –250, 125, and 62.5 μg/mL for 24, 48, and 72 hours, respectively). In addition, Fe_3O_4-NPs had a substantial lethal effect on A2780cp cells by inducing caspase-3 and -9-dependent apoptosis (intrinsic route). Palanisamy et al. [29] reported that the phytochemistry profile of concentrated *Sargassum polycystum* extracts contained variable secondary metabolites (including steroid, tannin, alkaloid, triterpenoid, and glycoside), etc. *S. polycystum* extract displayed cytotoxicity against colon HCT-116 and lung-A549 cells (IC_{50} values from 21.3 to 33.4 μg/mL). Palanisamy et al. [29] studied the anticancer properties of fucoidan from *Sargassum polycystum*. *S. polycystum* "Fucoidan" inhibited MCF-7 cells at a greater rate (90.4% at 150 μg/mL and IC_{50} of 50 μg/mL). Hamouda et al. [26] found that *Sargassum vulgare* produced Ag-NPs. Ag-NPs at varying doses showed antioxidant and anticancer activity on HepG-2, HCT-116, HeLa, and PC-3, with IC_{50} values of 50.4, 45.8, 78.4 and 100.3 μg/mL, respectively. Song et al. [59] isolated and purified 16 polysaccharide fractions (PF) from *Sargassum horneri*, *Scytosiphon lomentaria*, and *Undaria pinnatifida*. The antitumor activity of PF

Green seaweeds	Phytochemical constituents	Nanoparticles/crude extract	Cell lines Utilized	Bioactivity	References
Caulerpa racemosa	Protein, amino acids, carbohydrate	Au	Human lung cancer cells (H460)	Antimicrobial and anticancer	[34]
Caulerpa sertularioides	Protein, amino acids, carbohydrate	ZnO	*Artemia nauplii*	Antioxidant activities	[38]
Chaetomorpha sp	Protein, amino acids, carbohydrate, alkaloids, tannins, phenolic, flavonoids	Extract	MCF-7 and MDA-MB-231	Cytotoxic effect	[52]
Codium tomentosum	Fucoidan	Au	HEPG-2 cell line	Antitumoral activity	[58]
Cymodocea serrulata	Alkaloids, tannins, phenolic, flavonoids	Ag	A549 cells	antitumoral activity	[28]
Enteromorpha compressa	Alkaloids, tannins	Ag	Ehlrich ascites carcinoma (EAC) cells	Cytotoxicity	[30]
Gracilaria edulis	Alkaloids, tannins, phenolic, flavonoids	Au	Breast carcinoma cells (MDA-MB-231)	Antibacterial and cytotoxicity	[33]
Halimeda tuna	Protein, amino acids, carbohydrate, alkaloids, tannins, phenolic, flavonoids	Extract	Lung cancer cells (A549)	Cytotoxicity	[56]
Ulva lactuca	Protein, amino acids, carbohydrate, →4)-β-D-glucuronic acid	Phycocyanin	Liver and breast cancer cells	Antimicrobial and anticancer	[45]
Ulva rigida	Protein, amino acids, carbohydrate, alkaloids, tannins, phenolic, flavonoids	Extract	Human cervix adenocarcinoma (HeLa) cells	Cytotoxic effect	[25]

Table 1.
The metal and metal oxide nanoparticles synthesized using green seaweeds and its applications.

was tested against five different tumor cell lines, including A549, B16, HeLa, HepG2, and SH-SY5Y; findings revealed that various PF has differential antitumor activities against tested cells. Further, PF has increased the expression of tumor signaling caspase-3, caspase-8, caspase-9, and Bax, while decreasing expression of Bcl-2 and CDK-2, according to qRT-RCR findings [59]. Pugazhendhi et al. [43] produced magnesium oxide nanoparticles (MgO-NPs) from the marine brown algae *Sargassum wighitii*. MgO-NPs demonstrated dose-dependent cytotoxicity against A549 cells (IC_{50} = 37.5 μg/mL). Further, safety testing on peripheral blood mononuclear cells (PBMCs) revealed MgO-NPs to be non-toxic. Yunianta et al. [60] found that fucoidan isolated from *S. echinocarpum* was harmful to breast cancer cells (MCF-7) at 297 ppm. The extract caused apoptosis by 49.7, 72.0, and 89.3% after incubation for 24, 48, and 72 hours, respectively. Fucoidan raised MDA levels in MCF-7 cells, indicating anticancer activity via apoptosis-induced lipid peroxidation etc. Van Meerloo et al. [61] investigated the dose-dependent anticancer activity (MCF-7) of Au-NPs produced from *Sargassum officinalis*. Similarly, Wu et al. [62] found that fucoidans caused apoptosis in A549 cells by *Sargassum crassifolium*. Pal et al. [63] investigated the phytochemicals, antioxidants, and cytotoxic properties of *Sargassum prismaticum* in chloroform and methanol solvents. DPPH and ABTS assays were used to determine antioxidant activity; nevertheless, the methanolic extract outperformed the others. The methanolic extract showed the highest cell cytotoxicity (7.6 μg/mL), whereas the chloroform extract exhibited a higher cytotoxicity (9.6 μg/mL) against the U937 cell line. Kalaiselvi et al. [64] investigated the cytotoxicity of *Stoechospermum marginatum* ethanolic extract on HT-29 cells and found significant dose-dependent cytotoxicity, increased apoptotic cells, and decreased mitochondrial membrane potential. Further, Santhanam et al. [35] assessed the cytotoxicity of polysaccharides "fucoidan" isolated from *Turbinaria conoides.* The results revealed that fucoidan had a higher IC_{50} value for the MCF7 cell line (115.2 μg/mL) than the A549 cell line (396.46 μg/mL) after 24 hours of incubation. In contrast, fucoidan was discovered to be non-lethal to the L929 mouse fibroblast normal cell line. Similarly, Delma et al. [21] found that fucoidan from *Turbinaria conoides* reduced cell growth and promoted apoptosis in Mia PaCa-2 and PANC-1 human PC cell lines. At 100 g/mL, the extract inhibited the development of human aortic endothelial cell tubes, indicating substantial anti-angiogenic properties. Ermakova et al. [65] identified water-soluble polysaccharides from *Turbinaria ornata*, including laminaran, fucoidans, and ToF2. Polysaccharides and modified fucoidan derivatives (ToF2) were tested for anticancer efficacy against cancer cell lines including human colorectal, breast adenocarcinoma, and malignant melanoma. Fucoidan ToF2, an enzymatic hydrolysis derivative, inhibited colony formation in all cancer cells examined (**Table 2**).

7.3 Red seaweeds

Babu et al. [10] described Au-NPs from *Acanthophora spicifera*. *A. spicifera*-Au-NPs showed high cytotoxicity on HT-29, with an IC_{50} of 21.8 μg/mL. Janani et al. [67] studied the liposomal formulation of aqueous extract from *Amphiphora anceps*, a red seaweed species. The anticancer efficacy was examined using A549 cells. The NHA suppressed the cancer cells dose-dependently, with the maximum killing rate of 92% at 100 μg/mL. *In vivo* investigations in the zebrafish model revealed that *Amphiroa anceps*' HA and NHA had no teratogenic effects. Our analysis identified NHA as a promising cancer inhibitor with good biocompatibility up to 100 μg/mL. Viswanathan et al. [36] produced silver nanoparticles from *Champia parvula* extract, which showed good anticancer activity against A549 (IC_{50} = 21.5 μg/mL) and HT-29 cells (IC_{50} = 42.3 μg/mL).

DOI: http://dx.doi.org/10.5772/intechopen.1008314

Brown seaweed	Phytochemical constituents	Nanoparticles/ extract	Cell lines utilized	Bioactivity	References
Cystoseira myrica	Polyunsaturated fatty acids	Ag	Breast carcinoma cells (MCF-7)	Cytotoxicity	[27]
Sargassum echinocarpum	fucoidans	Fucoidans extract	Breast cancer cells (MCF-7)	Antitumor	[60]
Sargassum muticum	Alkaloids, tannins, phenolic, flavonoids	Fe3O4	Human cell lines for leukemia (Jurkat cells)	Antimicrobial and anticancer	[40]
Sargassum polycystum	Alkaloids, tannins, phenolic, flavonoids	Ag	human colon cancer (HT-29) cells	Antioxidant and anticancer	[29]
Sargassum vulgare	Alkaloids, tannins, phenolic, flavonoids	Ag-NPs	colon carcinoma (HCT-116)	Anticancer	[26]
Sargassum wightii	Sulfated polysaccharide	Au, MgO-NPs	Cervical cancer cell line, peripheral blood mononuclear cells	Antimicrobial and anticancer	[43]
Stoechospermum marginatum	Alkaloids, tannins, Phenolic, flavonoids	Ethanol Extract	HT-29 cells	Antioxidant, antimicrobial, and anticancer	[66]
Turbinaria conoides	alkaloids, tannins, phenolic, flavonoids	Ag and Au	*Artemia salina*	Antimicrobial and anticancer	[21, 35]
Turbinaria ornata	Polysaccharides, phenols, fucoidans	Ag and fucoidans extract	Retinoblastoma Y79 cell lines, malignant melanoma cell lines	Antimicrobial and anticancer	[31, 65]

Table 2.
Metal and metal oxide nanoparticles produced utilizing brown seaweeds and their applications.

El-Kassas and Mohamed [32] produced Au-NPs from the red algae *Corallina officinalis*. The Au-NPs had strong cytotoxic activity against MCF-7 cells, producing necrosis at high doses but having no effect at lower concentrations, as evidenced by a DNA fragmentation experiment. El-Rafie et al. [68] studied *Digenea simplex*, an Egyptian maritime red macroalgae, has a broad range of phytochemicals with distinct bioactivities. In antioxidant activity tests, *D. simplex* extract had IC_{50} values of 36.8 and 63.5% in DPPH and ABTS assays. This study suggests that *D. simplex* could enhance cytotoxic activity. Sudhakar et al. [69] isolated phycoerythrin pigment (PE) from *Gracilaria corticata*. PE showed significant antioxidant activity by DPPH scavenging (22.9%) and ferrous ion chelating capacity (26.0%). Additionally, the cytotoxicity of PE was investigated on SW620 and HCT-116 (colon cancer cells). The MTT experiment shows that adding 4.8 μg of PE reduces percent cell viability (42%) after 48 hours, SW 620 cell line. In HCT 116 cell line, increasing the concentration of PE stimulates cell growth for 24 hours but results in a 39% reduction in cell growth after 48 hours with 4.8 μg of PE. Hoang et al. [11] studied the biomass of red algae (*G. corticata*, *C. ocellatus*, and *P. perforate*) from marine sources contains significant proximate characteristics and nutritionally relevant minerals (Fe, Cu, Mg, and Zn). *In vitro* cytotoxicity test (MTT assay) showed that red algae methanol extract was highly hazardous to HeLa and MCF7 cells, followed by the hexane extract. Sivakumar et al. [49] produced copper oxide nanoparticles (CuO-NPs) from *Halymenia dilatata* aqueous extract. The HeLa cell line demonstrated considerable anticancer activity (IC_{50} value of 147.5 μg/mL) after 48 hours of treatment. Vinosha et al. [70] studied the bioactive characteristics of sulfated galactan (SGP) polysaccharides produced from the red macroalgae *Halymenia dilatata*. The isolated SGP showed significant cytotoxicity against MDA-MB-231 cells, with an IC_{50} of 75 μg/mL. Gomathy and Rushi [71] produced iron oxide nanoparticles (Fe_3O_4-NPs) from *Hypnea valentiae* and red seaweeds. Fe_3O_4-NPs are efficient enough against MDA-MB-231 (IC_{50} = 33.8 μg/mL) and A549 cells (IC_{50} = 66.7 μg/mL). Further, *H. valentiae*-Fe_3O_4-NPs successfully cause apoptotic activity by increasing ROS (reactive oxygen species) levels. In addition, At 34 μg/mL, *H. valentiae*-Fe_3O_4-NPs demonstrated substantial anticancer action by downregulating AKT and PI3K expression while upregulating PTEN expression (RT-PCR gene expression analysis). Molecular docking of *H. valentiae* drugs targeting the AKT/PI3K pathway proteins in breast cancer with aberrant mutations yielded favorable binding scores. In a study by Cholaraj and Venkatachalam [20], fucoidan isolated from *Padina boergesenii* was evaluated for antioxidant and anticancer properties. The highest antioxidant activity was observed in DPPH (76.7%), Reducing power (66.5%), ABTS (70.5%), H_2O_2 (59.9%), Total antioxidant scavenging (TAC) 68.92% at 1000 μg/mL with an IC_{50} value of 55.6, 59.7, 57.4, 64.4, 61.8 and 60.7, respectively. In addition, fucoidan – *P. boergesenii* inhibited HeLa cells by 54% at 40 μg/mL (IC_{50} = 38 μg/mL). Nikolova et al. [72] tested the anticancer potential of extracellular polysaccharide (ECP) obtained from *Porphyridium sordidum* using MCF-7 and MDA-MB231. Cell survival was dose and cell type dependent after 48 hours of administration. Ivanova et al. [73] separated extracellular polysaccharides (EPS) from *Porphyridium aerugineum*. *P. aerugineum* polysaccharide showed significant ABTS radical-scavenging activity, up to 55%. MCF-7 cells treated with 1000 μg/mL EPS for 72 hours exhibited the strongest cytotoxic impact, inhibiting tumor cell multiplication by over 70%. Arsianti et al. [74] found triterpenoid and alkaloid metabolites in the ethanol extract of *Eucheuma cottonii*. In addition, antioxidant activity (IC_{50} = 559.76 μg/mL) against DPPH. While the cytotoxicity test on A549 cells yielded (IC_{50} = 261.41 μg/mL). *Kappaphycus alvarezii* crude extract was evaluated on MCF-7 cells and administered to rats at a dose of 2000 mg/kg body weight for 60 days to assess chronic toxicity and heavy metal toxicity (**Table 3**) [19].

Red seaweeds	Phytochemical constituents	Nanoparticles/extract	Cell lines utilized	Bioactivity	Reference
Acanthophora spicifera	Alkaloids, tannins	Au	Human colon adenocarcinoma (HT-29) cells	Antimicrobial and anticancer	[10]
Amphiphora anceps	Alkaloids, tannins	Aqueous extract	A549 cells	Anticancer activity	[67]
Champia parvula	Alkaloids, tannins, phenolic, flavonoids	Se at Zn NPs, Au-NPs, Ag-NPs, extract	A549, MCF-7, HT-29 and HeLa cell lines	Antimicrobial, antitumor activity, and apoptosis	[36]
Corallina officinalis	Alkaloids, tannins, phenolic, flavonoids	Au	Human breast cancer (MCF-7)	Antimicrobial and anticancer	[32]
Digenea simplex	Alkaloids, tannins, phenolic, flavonoids	ChlE-NS	Human colon cancer cell line	Cytotoxic and antioxidant activities	[68]
Eucheuma cottonii	Triterpenoid and alkaloid metabolites	Ethanol extract	A-549	Cytotoxic and antioxidant activities	[74]
Gracilaria corticata	Phycoerythrin	Phycoerythrin extract	SW 620, HCT 116 cell line	Antimicrobial activity	[69]
Gracilaria verrucosa	Alkaloids, tannins, phenolic, flavonoids	Au	HEK-293 cells	Antitumor activity	[37]
Halymenia dilatata	Alkaloids, tannins	Cu	HeLa cell line	Antimicrobial and anticancer	[49]
Hypnea valentiae	sulfated polysaccharide, carrageenan	Au	A549 cells	Antimicrobial and anticancer	[71]
Kappaphycus alvarezii	Alkaloids, tannins, phenolic, flavonoids	Crude extract	MCF-7 cells	Antitumor activity	[19]
Padina boergesenii	Fucoidans	Fucoidans extract	human cervical carcinoma cells (HeLa)	Cytotoxic and antioxidant activities	[20]
Porphyridium aerugineum	Extracellular polysaccharide	Polysaccharide extract	MCF-7 (breast cancer) and HeLa	Anticancer	[73]

Red seaweeds	Phytochemical constituents	Nanoparticles/extract	Cell lines utilized	Bioactivity	Reference
Porphyridium sordidum	Extracellular polysaccharide	Polysaccharide extract	MCF-7,MDA-MB231	Anticancer	[72]
Turbinaria ornata	Fucoidans	Fucoidans extract	Malignant melanoma cell lines	Antitumor activity	[65]

Table 3.
Applications of metal and metal oxide nanoparticles produced from red seaweeds.

8. Conclusion

This review paper focuses on the diverse applications of metal and metal oxide nanoparticles generated from seaweeds. Seaweeds have attracted a lot of attention in nanoparticle synthesis research because of their potential applications in a variety of sectors, including medicine. Further, this article addresses nanoparticle formation, characterization, and application mechanisms. This report also discusses the extraction procedure, solvents used, phytochemicals involved, and variables affecting nanoparticle production. Bioactive nanoparticles derived from marine seaweeds offer a wide range of biological uses, the most prominent of which being drug delivery and cancer treatment.

Acknowledgements

The authors are grateful to the management of JJ College of Arts and Science (A), Pudukkottai for providing facilities for this study.

Conflicts of interest

The authors declare no conflict of interest.

Author details

Pitchai Palaniappan[1*], Kannaiah Surendirakumar[2], Manoharan Ravi[3] and Ramar Ramesh[1]

1 Department of Biochemistry, JJ College of Arts and Science (Autonomous), (Affiliated to Bharathidasan University, Tiruchirappalli), Pudukkottai, Tamilnadu, India

2 Department of Microbiology, JJ College of Arts and Science (Autonomous), (Affiliated to Bharathidasan University, Tiruchirappalli), Pudukkottai, Tamilnadu, India

3 Department of Biochemistry, University of Madras, Guindy Campus, Chennai, Tamilnadu, India

*Address all correspondence to: biopalani82@gmail.com

References

[1] Bayda S, Adeel M, Tuccinardi T, Cordani M, Rizzolio F. The history of nanoscience and nanotechnology: From chemical–physical applications to nanomedicine. Molecules. 2019;**25**(1):112

[2] Biris-Dorhoi ES, Michiu D, Pop CR, Rotar AM, Tofana M, Pop OL, et al. Macroalgae—A sustainable source of chemical compounds with biological activities. Nutrients. 2020;**12**(10):3085

[3] Venkatesan J, Anil S, Kim SK, Shim MS. Seaweed polysaccharide-based nanoparticles: Preparation and applications for drug delivery. Polymers. 2016;**8**(2):30

[4] Arockiya ARF, Parthiban C, Ganesh Kumar V, Anantharaman P. Biosynthesis of antibacterial gold nanoparticles using brown alga, *Stoechospermum marginatum* (kützing). Spectrochimica Acta, Part A: Molecular and Biomolecular Spectroscopy. 2012;**99**:166-173

[5] Bhardwaj B, Singh P, Kumar A, Kumar S, Budhwar V. Eco-friendly greener synthesis of nanoparticles. Advanced Pharmaceutical Bulletin. 2020;**10**(4):566

[6] Ying S, Guan Z, Ofoegbu PC, Clubb P, Rico C, He F, et al. Green synthesis of nanoparticles: Current developments and limitations. Environmental Technology & Innovation. 2022;**26**:102336

[7] Jha S, Rani R, Singh S. Biogenic zinc oxide nanoparticles and their biomedical applications: A review. Journal of Inorganic and Organometallic Polymers and Materials. 2023;**33**(6):1437-1452

[8] Chan SS, Low SS, Chew KW, Ling TC, Rinklebe J, Juan JC, et al. Prospects and environmental sustainability of phyconanotechnology: A review on algae-mediated metal nanoparticles synthesis and mechanism. Environmental Research. 2022;**212**:113140

[9] Agena R, de Jesús C-SA, Hernández-Sánchez H, Jaramillo-Flores ME. Pro-apoptotic activity of bioactive compounds from seaweeds: Promising sources for developing novel anticancer drugs. Marine Drugs. 2023;**21**(3):182

[10] Babu B, Palanisamy S, Vinosha M, Anjali R, Kumar P, Pandi B, et al. Bioengineered gold nanoparticles from marine seaweed *Acanthophora spicifera* for pharmaceutical uses: Antioxidant, antibacterial, and anticancer activities. Bioprocess and Biosystems Engineering. 2020;**43**:2231-2242

[11] Hoang TV, Alfarraj S, Alharbi SA. An investigation on antimicrobial and anticancer competence of macro red algae under in vitro condition. Environmental Research. 2024;**252**:119026

[12] Siegel RL, Giaquinto AN, Jemal A. Cancer statistics, 2024. CA: A Cancer Journal for Clinicians. 2024;**74**(1):12-49

[13] Leiter A, Veluswamy RR, Wisnivesky JP. The global burden of lung cancer: Current status and future trends. Nature Reviews Clinical Oncology. 2023;**20**(9):624-639

[14] Mathur P, Sathishkumar K, Chaturvedi M, Das P, Sudarshan KL, Santhappan S, et al. Cancer statistics, 2020: Report from national cancer registry programme, India. JCO Global Oncology. 2020;**6**(6):1063-1075

[15] Wolf A, Oeffinger KC, Shih TY, Walter LC, Church TR, Fontham ET, et al. Screening for Lung Cancer: 2023 Guideline Update from the American Cancer Society. CA: A Cancer Journal for Clinicians; 2023

[16] Xia C, Dong X, Li H, Cao M, Sun D, He S, et al. Cancer statistics in China and United States, 2022: Profiles, trends, and determinants. Chinese Medical Journal. 2022;**135**(05):584-590

[17] Khaltaev N, Axelrod S. Global lung cancer mortality trends and lifestyle modifications: Preliminary analysis. Chinese Medical Journal. 2020;**133**(13):1526-1532

[18] Zang EA, Wynder EL. Differences in lung cancer risk between men and women: Examination of the evidence. JNCI: Journal of the National Cancer Institute. 1996;**88**(3-4):183-192

[19] Chang VS, Okechukwu PN, Teo SS. The properties of red seaweed (*Kappaphycus alvarezii*) and its effect on mammary carcinogenesis. Biomedicine & Pharmacotherapy. 2017;**87**:296-301

[20] Cholaraj R, Venkatachalam R. Investigation of antioxidant and anticancer potential of fucoidan (in-vitro & in-silico) from brown seaweed *Padina boergesenii*. Algal Research. 2024;**79**:103442

[21] Delma CR, Somasundaram ST, Srinivasan GP, Khursheed M, Bashyam MD, Aravindan N. Fucoidan from *Turbinaria conoides*: A multifaceted 'deliverable' to combat pancreatic cancer progression. International Journal of Biological Macromolecules. 2015;**74**:447-457

[22] Güler C, Güner A, Yavaşoğlu NÜ. Cytotoxicity and anti-angiogenic potential of a macro alga, *Ulva rigida* C. Agardh (green alga) from Izmir Bay (Turkey). Biology Bulletin. 2023;**50**(Suppl 3):S261-S269

[23] Püsküllüoğlu M, Michalak I. An ocean of possibilities: A review of marine organisms as sources of nanoparticles for cancer care. Nanomedicine. 2022;**17**(22):1695-1719

[24] Soenen S, Bonomi AG, Lemmens SG, Scholte J, Thijssen MA, Van Berkum F, et al. Relatively high-protein or 'low-carb' energy-restricted diets for body weight loss and body weight maintenance? Physiology & Behavior. 2012;**107**(3):374-380

[25] Mukherjee A, Sarkar D, Sasmal S. A review of green synthesis of metal nanoparticles using algae. Frontiers in Microbiology. 2021;**12**:693899

[26] Hamouda RA, Abdel-Hamid MS, Hagagy N, Nofal AM. The potent effect of selenium nanoparticles: Insight into the antifungal activity and preservation of postharvest strawberries from gray mold diseases. Journal of the Science of Food and Agriculture. 2024;**104**(11):6756-6768

[27] Mohamed RM, Fawzy EM, Shehab RA, Abdel-Salam MO, Salah El Din RA, Abd El Fatah HM. Production, characterization, and cytotoxicity effects of silver nanoparticles from Brown alga (*Cystoseira myrica*). Journal of Nanotechnology. 2022;**2022**(1):6469090, 1-11

[28] Palaniappan P, Sathishkumar G, Sankar R. Fabrication of nano-silver particles using *Cymodocea serrulata* and its cytotoxicity effect against human lung cancer A549 cells line. Spectrochimica Acta Part A: Molecular and Biomolecular Spectroscopy. 2015;**138**:885-890

[29] Palanisamy S, Vinosha M, Marudhupandi T, Rajasekar P,

Prabhu NM. Isolation of fucoidan from Sargassum polycystum brown algae: Structural characterization, *in vitro* antioxidant and anticancer activity. International Journal of Biological Macromolecules. 2017;**102**:405-412

[30] Ramkumar VS, Pugazhendhi A, Gopalakrishnan K, Sivagurunathan P, Saratale GD, Dung TN, et al. Biofabrication and characterization of silver nanoparticles using aqueous extract of seaweed *Enteromorpha compressa* and its biomedical properties. Biotechnology Reports. 2017;**14**:1-7

[31] Remya RR, Rajasree SR, Suman TY, Aranganathan L, Gayathri S, Gobalakrishnan M, et al. Laminarin based AgNPs using brown seaweed *Turbinaria ornata* and its induction of apoptosis in human retinoblastoma Y79 cancer cell lines. Materials Research Express. 2018;**5**(3):035403

[32] El-Kassas HY, Mohamed LA. Bioremediation of the textile waste effluent by *Chlorella vulgaris*. Egyptian Journal of Aquatic Research. 2014;**40**(3):301-308

[33] Mohanta YK, Mishra AK, Nayak D, Patra B, Bratovcic A, Avula SK, et al. Exploring dose-dependent cytotoxicity profile of Gracilaria edulis-mediated green synthesized silver nanoparticles against MDA-MB-231 breast carcinoma. Oxidative Medicine and Cellular Longevity. 2022;**2022**(1):3863138

[34] Palaniappan P, Subramani P, Selvarajan R, Sankar R, Vilwanathan R, Sibanda T. Green synthesis of gold nanoparticles (AuNPs) using *Caulerpa racemosa* and evaluation of its antibacterial and cytotoxic activity against human lung cancer cell line. Arab Journal of Basic and Applied Sciences. 2022;**29**(1):351-362

[35] Santhanam RC, Yacoob SA, Venkatraman A. *In vitro* cytotoxicity assay of Fucoidan extracted from *Turbinaria conoides* against cancer cell lines MCF7, A549, and normal cell line L929. Brazilian Journal of Pharmaceutical Sciences. 2022;**58**:e19542

[36] Viswanathan S, Palaniyandi T, Shanmugam R, Karunakaran S, Pandi M, Wahab MR, et al. Synthesis, characterization, cytotoxicity, and antimicrobial studies of green synthesized silver nanoparticles using red seaweed *Champia parvula*. Biomass Conversion and Biorefinery. 2024;**14**(6):7387-7400

[37] Chellapandian C, Ramkumar B, Puja P, Shanmuganathan R, Pugazhendhi A, Kumar P. Gold nanoparticles using red seaweed Gracilaria verrucosa: Green synthesis, characterization and biocompatibility studies. Process Biochemistry. 2019;**80**:58-63

[38] Solomon J, Palanisamy S, Ravichandran A, Rajasekar P, Kannan SM, Malaikozhundan B, et al. Characterization and investigation of biofabricated ZnO nanoparticles using Caulerpa sertularioides for antioxidant and antibacterial purposes. Inorganic Chemistry Communications. 2024;**165**:112549

[39] Chandran M, Yuvaraj D, Christudhas L, Ramesh KV. Bio synthesis of iron nanoparticles using the brown seaweed, *Dictyota dicotoma*. Indian Journal of Biotechnology. 2016;**12**(12):112

[40] Namvar F, Amini E, Mahdavi M. Cytotoxic effect of magnetic iron oxide nanoparticles coated with seaweed aqueous extract against ovarian cancer cells. KAUMS Journal (FEYZ). 2015;**19**(2):94-101

[41] Palaniyandi T, Baskar GVB, Viswanathan S, Abdul Wahab MR, Govindaraj MK, Sivaji A, et al. Biosynthesis of iron nanoparticles using brown algae *Spatoglossum asperum* and its antioxidant and anticancer activities through *in vitro* and in silico studies. Particulate Science and Technology. 2023;**41**(7):916-929

[42] Fouda A, Eid AM, Abdel-Rahman MA, El-Belely EF, Awad MA, Hassan SE, et al. Enhanced antimicrobial, cytotoxicity, larvicidal, and repellence activities of brown algae, *Cystoseira crinita*-mediated green synthesis of magnesium oxide nanoparticles. Frontiers in Bioengineering and Biotechnology. 2022;**10**:849921

[43] Pugazhendhi A, Prabhu R, Muruganantham K, Shanmuganathan R, Natarajan S. Anticancer, antimicrobial and photocatalytic activities of green synthesized magnesium oxide nanoparticles (MgONPs) using aqueous extract of *Sargassum wightii*. Journal of Photochemistry and Photobiology B: Biology. 2019;**190**:86-97

[44] Fawcett D, Verduin JJ, Shah M, Sharma SB, Poinern GE. A review of current research into the biogenic synthesis of metal and metal oxide nanoparticles via marine algae and seagrasses. Journal of Nanoscience. 2017;**2017**(1):8013850

[45] Thanh TT, Ngo QV, Nguyen TT, Nguyen AN, Quach TT, Dang LV, et al. Ulvan from green seaweed *Ulva lactuca*: Optimization of ultrasound-assisted extraction, structure, and cytotoxic activity. Journal of Carbohydrate Chemistry. 2023;**42**(1-3):92-111

[46] Abdel-Raouf N, Al-Enazi NM, Ibraheem IB, Alharbi RM, Alkhulaifi MM. Biosynthesis of silver nanoparticles by using of the marine brown alga *Padina pavonia* and their characterization. Saudi Journal of Biological Sciences. 2019;**26**(6):1207-1215

[47] Abboud Y, Saffaj T, Chagraoui A, El Bouari A, Brouzi K, Tanane O, et al. Biosynthesis, characterization and antimicrobial activity of copper oxide nanoparticles (CONPs) produced using brown alga extract (*Bifurcaria bifurcata*). Applied Nanoscience. 2014;**4**:571-576

[48] Deepak P, Amutha V, Birundha R, Sowmiya R, Kamaraj C, Balasubramanian V, et al. Facile green synthesis of nanoparticles from brown seaweed *Sargassum wightii* and its biological application potential. Advances in Natural Sciences: Nanoscience and Nanotechnology. 2018a;**9**(3):035019

[49] Sivakumar SR, Manimaran K, Govindasamy M, Alzahrani FM, Alsaiari NS. Green synthesis and characterization of CuO nanoparticles using *Halymenia dilatata* extract and its evaluation of antimicrobial, anticancer activity. Biomass Conversion and Biorefinery. 2023;**14**:27623-27632

[50] Kavaz D, Umar H, Zimuto T. Biosynthesis of gold nanoparticles using *Scytosiphon lomentaria* (Brown algae) and *Spyridia filamentosa* (red algae) from Kyrenia region and evaluation of their antimicrobial and antioxidant activity. Hacettepe Journal of Biology and Chemistry. 2019;**47**(4):367-382

[51] Rajeshkumar S, Parameswari RP, Jayapriya J, Tharani M, Ali H, Aljarba NH, et al. [Retracted] apoptotic and antioxidant activity of gold nanoparticles synthesized using marine brown seaweed: An *in vitro* study. BioMed Research International. 2022;**2022**(1):5746761

[52] Nova P, Gomes AM, Costa-Pinto AR. It comes from the sea: Macroalgae-derived bioactive compounds with anti-cancer potential. Critical Reviews in Biotechnology. 2024;**44**(3):462-476

[53] Ragunath C, Madeshwaran K, Paulraj D, Murugesan S, Venkatachalam R. Biosynthesis and characterization of silver nanoparticles using polysaccharides from *Caulerpa racemosa* and evaluation of their antioxidant, antibacterial, and anticancer activities. Next Nanotechnology. 2024;**6**:100088

[54] Quach TT, Nguyen NT, Yuguchi Y, Dang LV, Van Ngo Q, Thanh TT. Structure, anticoagulant and cytotoxic activity of a sulfated polysaccharide from green seaweed *Chaetomorpha linum*. Natural Product Research. 2024;**38**(4):555-562

[55] Akter M, Sikder MT, Rahman MM, Ullah AA, Hossain KF, Banik S, et al. A systematic review on silver nanoparticles-induced cytotoxicity: Physicochemical properties and perspectives. Journal of Advanced Research. 2018;**9**:1-6

[56] Husni A, Gazali M, Nurjanah N, Syafitri R, Matin A, Zuriat Z. Cytotoxic activity of green seaweed Halimeda tuna methanolic extract against lung cancer cells. Journal of Multidisciplinary Applied Natural Science. 2024;**4**(1):16-29

[57] Alshehri MA, Panneerselvam C. Green synthesis of graphene-based derivatives from *Ulva lactuca* extract: Characterization and biomedical applications. Journal of Industrial and Engineering Chemistry. 2024;**141**:554-567

[58] González-Ballesteros N, Maietta I, Rey-Méndez R, Rodríguez-Argüelles MC, Lastra-Valdor M, Cavazza A, et al. Gold nanoparticles synthesized by an aqueous extract of Codium tomentosum as potential antitumoral enhancers of gemcitabine. Marine Drugs. 2022;**21**(1):1-19

[59] Song L, Niu Y, Chen R, Ju H, Liu Z, Zhang B, et al. A comparative analysis of the anti-tumor activity of sixteen polysaccharide fractions from three large brown seaweed, *Sargassum horneri*, *Scytosiphon lomentaria*, and *Undaria pinnatifida*. Marine Drugs. 2024;**22**(7):316

[60] Yunianta Y, Laeliocattleya RA, Wulan SN, Risjani Y. Fucoidan extract from brown seaweed (*Sargassum echinocarpum*): Molecular weight, elemental composition, selectivity and anticancer activity against breast cancer cells. Natural Product Research. 2024;**3**:1-9

[61] Van Meerloo J, Kaspers GJ, Cloos J. Cell sensitivity assays: The MTT assay. Cancer Cell Culture: Methods and Protocols. 2011;**731**:237-245

[62] Wu TC, Hong YH, Tsai YH, Hsieh SL, Huang RH, Kuo CH, et al. Degradation of *Sargassum crassifolium* fucoidan by ascorbic acid and hydrogen peroxide, and compositional, structural, and *in vitro* anti-lung cancer analyses of the degradation products. Marine Drugs. 2020;**18**(6):334

[63] Pal S, Soni A, Patel N, Sharma P, Siddiqi NJ, Fatima S, et al. Phytochemical profiling, antioxidant potential and cytotoxic activity of *Sargassum prismaticum* extracts: Implications for therapeutic applications. Natural Product Research. 2024:1-7

[64] Kalaiselvi L, Sriram P, Gokulakannan R, Parthiban M, Kannan TA, Preetha SP, et al. Chemopreventive effect of *Stoechospermum marginatum* against

experimental colon carcinogenesis induced by 1, 2-dimethyl hydrazine. Indian Journal of Animal Research. 2022;**56**(4):460-467

[65] Ermakova SP, Menshova RV, Anastyuk SD, Zakharenko AM, Thinh PD, Ly BM, et al. Structure, chemical and enzymatic modification, and anticancer activity of polysaccharides from the brown alga *Turbinaria ornata*. Journal of Applied Phycology. 2016;**28**:2495-2505

[66] Sarangi NV, Harini AB, Rajkumar R, Veeramuthu A. Evaluation of chemical constituents of Stoechospermum marginatum and its potential for antioxidant and antimicrobial activity. Biomass Conversion and Biorefinery. 2023;**22**:1-12

[67] Janani G, Girigoswami A, Deepika B, Udayakumar S, Girigoswami K. Unveiling the role of nano-formulated red algae extract in cancer management. Molecules. 2024;**29**(9):2077

[68] El-Rafie HM, Hasan EA, Zahran MK. Enhancement of cytotoxic and antioxidant activities of *Digenea simplex* chloroform extract using the nanosuspension technique. Bioprocess and Biosystems Engineering. 2023;**46**(2):279-296

[69] Sudhakar MP, Dharani G, Paramasivam A. Evaluation of antimicrobial, antioxidant and cytotoxicity potential of R-phycoerythrin extracted from *Gracilaria corticata* seaweed. Current Research in Green and Sustainable Chemistry. 2023;**6**:100352

[70] Vinosha M, Palanisamy S, Jeneeta S, Rajasekar P, Marudhupandi T, Karthikeyan M, et al. Antibacterial, anticancer and antioxidant effects of sulfated galactan from *Halymenia dilatata*: *In vitro* and *in vivo* analysis. Food. Bioscience. 2024;**60**:104420

[71] Gomathy G, Rushi KB. Thin film flow dynamics and heat transfer enhancement in porous media: Shape-dependent behavior of Al_2O_3 nanoparticles. Numerical Heat Transfer, Part A: Applications. 2024;**1**:1-18

[72] Nikolova B, Semkova S, Tsoneva I, Antov G, Ivanova J, Vasileva I, et al. Characterization and potential antitumor effect of a heteropolysaccharide produced by the red alga Porphyridium sordidum. Engineering in Life Sciences. 2019;**19**(12):978-985

[73] Ivanova JG, Toshkova-Yotova TS, Toshkova RA, Deleva VR, Georgieva AK, Gigova LG. Antioxidant and anticancer potential of extracellular polysaccharide from *Porphyridium aerugineum* (Rhodophyta). Fermentation. 2024;**10**(5):259

[74] Arsianti A, Kurniawan G, Tejaputri NA, Qorina F, Fithrotunnisa Q, Azizah NN, et al. Phytochemical profile, antioxidant activity and cell line study of marine red macroalgae Eucheuma cottonii on lung A-549 cancer cells. Pharmacognosy Journal. 2020;**12**(2):276-281

Chapter 5

Cytotoxicity Is the Key Test for *In Vitro* Toxicity

Terenteva Ekaterina Olegovna, Khashimova Zaynat Sattarovna, Khamidova Umida Bakhriddin Kizi, Umarova Mukaddas Rustamovna, Tosheva Nigora Arziyevna, Alimukhamedova Orzigul Bakhrievna and Azimova Shakhnoz Sadikovna

Abstract

Currently, a lot of new chemical compounds are registered in the world, some of them are used in various fields of medicine, pharmaceuticals or related fields. In this case, each of the introduced chemical compounds must be assessed toxicologically. *In vitro* cell models are used to elucidate the mechanisms of differentiation and proliferation, interaction of cells with the environment, adaptation, aging, biological activity, malignant transformation, for the diagnosis and treatment of hereditary diseases, and as test objects when testing new pharmacological substances. The review presents the advantages of using cell models, provides methods for studying the cytotoxic effects of target agents, and discusses the system for controlling the contamination of materials. In addition, the necessity to search for new cytostatics in the context of a steady trend of growth in new cases of cancer and the imperfections of existing anticancer drugs is discussed, and studies of the cytotoxicity of a number of promising tetrahydroisoquinolines, their structural-functional relationship, the type of triggering of cell death and the mechanism of manifestation of cytotoxicity are presented.

Keywords: cell models, cytotoxic effects, tetrahydroisoquinolines, structural-functional relationship, cytostatics

1. Introduction

Currently, about 700 thousand new chemical compounds are registered in the world. Among them, an average of 15% are used in various fields of medicine, pharmaceuticals or related fields. According to the current situation throughout the world, each of the introduced chemical compounds must be assessed toxicologically. Methods for studying substances *in vitro* make it possible to solve ethical problems associated with the massive use and death of experimental animals. Also, the time required for preliminary research of new chemical compounds and the costs at the stage of their preclinical testing are significantly reduced. The main advantage of *in vitro* models is their easy reproducibility, the ability to automate and conduct research directly on human cells, which allows the obtained results to be interpreted in terms of the whole organism [1]. Cell lines are used to solve such general biological problems as elucidating the mechanisms of differentiation and proliferation, interaction of cells with the environment, adaptation, aging, biological activity, malignant transformation, etc. [2, 3]. Cell culture is an integral part of tissue culture and tissue engineering technology because it defines the basis for growing cells and maintaining them in a viable state ex vivo. Cell lines are used for the diagnosis and treatment of hereditary diseases, and as test objects when testing new pharmacological substances. It has now been revealed that the response of cells that are protective in nature and ensure adaptation of the body to the influence of various unfavorable factors (for example, toxic agents) occurs through a single fundamental mechanism, which in turn leads to similar changes at the morphological and molecular levels [4]. The response mechanism is damage to cell membranes, increased peroxidation of membrane lipids, suppression of the activity of a number of cellular dehydrogenases and glutathione metabolism enzymes. The cellular response can occur regardless of the chemical structure of the toxic substance and the method of assessing cytotoxicity; depends little on the tissue and species origin of the cultured cells [5]. This universal nature of stress reactions makes the use of *in vitro* models very promising for assessing the viability and metabolic changes of cells not only when exposed to chemical compounds, but also identifying the influence of physical and biological factors (electromagnetic fields, viruses, tissue fluids of patients).

2. Cancer cell panels

The first panel of cancer cell lines was collected and tested in 1990 at the National Cancer Institute 60, USA (NCI-60). It consisted of 60 cancer cell lines representing nine major tumor types. A few years later, the Japan Cancer Research Foundation developed its own panel of 39 cancer cell lines, also based on nine types of tumors. Although the cell culture set replicated the 30 cell lines used in NCI-60, it also included six types of gastric cancer cells due to the prevalence of this type of cancer in the Japanese. The large number of cell lines has not only contributed to the accumulation of a large amount of information, but has also led to confusion about the origin of some cell lines and the development of new analytical methodologies for the integration of high-throughput data. In this regard, the American Standards Association ASN-0002 has developed a standardized protocol and database available for searching and authenticating human cell lines with the possibility of specific purposes [6].

Currently, *in vitro* testing systems are included in the screening program of Cancer Chemotherapy National Service Center, USA-CCNSC, as well as National Institutes of Health, USA-NIH, WHO Cancer Research Centers (Belgium); The European Partnership for Alternative Approaches to Animal Testing-EPAA; Japanese Center for the Validation of Alternative Methods-JaCVAM and other countries. Since 2007, the Office of the National Cancer Institute (NCI) of Complementary and Alternative Medicine (OCCAM) together with the Cancer Institute of the Chinese Academy of Chinese Medical Sciences (CICACMS), as well as the Institutes of the Chinese

DOI: http://dx.doi.org/10.5772/intechopen.1008310

Academy of Sciences and the Chinese Medical Academy of Sciences, conducts extensive screening of antitumor compounds on various sarcoma cell lines *in vitro* [7].

Moreover, the requirements of the legislation of these countries require the conduct of such studies in accordance with Good Laboratory Practice (GLP) standards [8]. GLP are the principles on the basis of which the planning and conduct of preclinical studies, the preparation of protocols and the preparation of research reports are carried out. GLP standards were first used in practice by the US Federal Food and Drug Administration back in the late 70s of the twentieth century [8]. Compliance with GLP rules ensures the reliability of research results and their reproducibility.

3. Assays for studying toxicity *in vitro*

To identify the cytotoxic effect of biologically active substances against cell lines, various research methods are used. These include microscopic equipment that allows visual detection of morphological changes under the influence of introduced agents, the use of special electronic devices—a particle counter or a cell counter with radioactive substances previously included in them. In addition, methods for quantifying total protein with incorporated chromogenic dyes or by measuring the metabolic activity of cellular enzymes are being actively used.

Previously, the most common test for detecting cell activity was the method of incorporating 3H-thymidine into cellular DNA. However, this analysis, despite its high sensitivity, is very labor-intensive, since it requires removal of excess unincorporated label using a certain method of cell treatment before measurement.

Another simple and accessible method is cell counting in a Goryaev chamber using dyes. For example, trypan blue is a dye that practically does not penetrate the cell membrane of intact cells [9]. An increase in the permeability of the cell membrane from damage by any toxicant leads to an increase in the amount of dye that enters the cell and binds to the components of the cytoplasm. As marker of lysosomal activity method for determining cell activity is the use of a neutral red dye. This test was first developed by Dr. Ellen Borenfreund in 1984. In this method, living cells incorporate neutral red into their lysosomes and Golgi apparatus. Dying cells are unable to turn on neutral red. Thus, loss of neutral red uptake corresponds to loss of cell viability [10].

Another intravital water-soluble stain is resazurin, which has been used since the 1950s to assess bacterial and yeast contamination of body fluids and milk. This detection method is based on the ability of living cells to reduce blue non-fluorescent resazurin to pink fluorescent resorufin, which can be determined colorimetrically or fluorimetrically. Resazurin is reduced by a wide range of enzymes: mitochondrial dehydrogenases, cytochromes and cell cytoplasmic dehydrogenases.

In 1956, the first paper was published on the use of tetrazolium salt as an indicator of cell viability. The method was based on the discovery that living cells are capable of reducing tetrazolium salts into intensely colored formazan derivatives. This conversion process requires the participation of mitochondria, which are inactivated within a few minutes after cell death. Therefore, this method is an excellent tool for identifying living and dead cells. However, the use of tetrazolium salts (MTT, MTS) irreversibly stopped cell proliferation, since it required cell destruction for dye release, and thus made it impossible to extend the incubation to increase sensitivity or continue cell cultivation. All this led to the appearance of tetrazolium salts with soluble reduction products (XTT-2,3-bis-(2-methoxy-4-nitro-5-sulfophenyl)-2H-tetrazolium-5-carboxanilide and WST-2-(2-methoxy-4-nitropentyl)-3-(4-nitropentyl)-5-(2,4-disulfophenyl)-2H-tetrazolium), which eliminated the associated disadvantages [11].

The sulforhodamine B (SRB) assay is used for cell density determination, based on the measurement of cellular protein content. After an incubation period, cell monolayers are fixed with 10% (wt/vol) trichloroacetic acid and stained for 30 min, after which the excess dye is removed by washing repeatedly with 1% (vol/vol) acetic acid. The protein-bound dye is dissolved in Tris base solution for OD determination at 510 nm using a microplate reader. The results are linear over a 20-fold range of cell numbers and the sensitivity is comparable to those of fluorometric methods. The SRB assay is therefore an efficient and highly cost-effective method for screening [12].

Basic toxic effects can also be determined using a test with the enzyme lactate dehydrogenase, which is a marker of membrane integrity. It is a cytosolic enzyme that is involved in the reversible conversion of pyruvate to lactate and is found in most tissues of the body. Lactate dehydrogenase is released into the culture medium from damage to the cytoplasmic membrane of cells [13].

For studying cytotoxic objects, a method based on double fluorescent staining of cells with Annexin V Alexa Fluor 488 and propidium iodide (PI) is also used to assess the number of living, apoptotic and late apoptotic cells. Annexin V binds specifically and with high affinity to phosphatidylserine appearing on the surface of apoptotic cells. PI penetrates only into dead cells and binds to the minor groove of DNA. Cells that are at a late stage of apoptosis or have already died will be positive for both markers (AnnV+PI+). This occurs due to the fact that membrane asymmetry is already disrupted, starting from the early stages of apoptosis, and in the later stages of apoptosis, the cellular and nuclear membranes become permeable to DNA-binding dyes.

Various research departments are working to develop methods for assessing cell proliferation that combine the study of several targets simultaneously. For example, BioMedica has created a dual-labeled assay with EZ4U and a radioactive nucleotide. The method combines the thymidine and MTT methods; it does not require removing the culture medium before or after adding a chromogenic substrate, dissolving or treating the cells. The chromophore used in the analysis is non-toxic [14].

Today, the main trends in gene-directed therapy for malignant diseases include strategies to suppress the overexpression of oncogenes and restore the expression of tumor suppressor genes, including compounds of plant origin and their synthetic derivatives. The possibility of inhibiting gene expression was first shown in [15–17] and was further developed within the framework of the idea of regulating the expression of genes involved in carcinogenesis under the influence of antisense [18] and gene-targeted oligonucleotides [19]. *In vitro* cell models of cancer cells make it possible to quickly, accurately and effectively identify the target for the manifestation of the cytotoxic effects of the studied cytostatics.

Thus, the large number of tests currently available for high-throughput screening of chemical compounds is certainly not limited to the methods listed above. To select a particular screening method, it is necessary to take into account the possibility of interaction of the test compounds with components of the test kit or with cells that can distort data on cell viability, the sensitivity of the method, the duration and cost of the test.

4. Detection of microbiological contamination in cell cultures

The active use of cell cultures in basic research and biotechnological production makes it necessary to develop a system for strict control of material contamination. There is always a risk of contamination of the cell lines with eukaryotic cells of other lines, as well as microorganisms, including fungi, viruses, and bacteria. Of particular importance is the contamination of cells with mycoplasmas, which does not manifest itself visually [20–22]. Cell cultures of all types, originating from various eukaryotic organisms (mammals, birds, reptiles, fish, insects and plants), are susceptible to contamination by mycoplasmas. Mycoplasmas are the collective name for the smallest representatives of the Mollicutes class, lacking a bacterial cell wall and capable of independent reproduction [23]. Contamination with mycoplasma can remain undetected for a long time; changes become visible only with a high multiplicity of infection [20, 22]. The most pronounced effect of contamination is the complete loss of the cell line due to the growth of microorganisms and, accordingly, irreversible deterioration of the cells. Depending on the type of mycoplasma, type of cell line and culture conditions, a variety of cytopathic reactions can be recorded. For example, chromatin condensation, the appearance of "leopard" cells, the occurrence of chromosomal aberrations, suppression of cell division, and inhibition of cell line growth may be observed [24, 25]. The main reason for these changes is the interference of mycoplasma in cellular metabolism, competitive absorption of nutritional components and the release of bacterial toxins, protein, DNA, and RNA degradation enzymes [20, 25].

Currently, several methods are used to detect mycoplasma infection of cells. The most effective way to detect mycoplasma contamination today is considered to be the use of polymerase chain reaction (PCR) [26, 27]. PCR options allow the detection of DNA or RNA of mycoplasmas. Oligonucleotides are usually used as primers to amplify variable regions of 16S rDNA or rRNA, as well as sequences of 16-23S intergenic regions. In some cases, with a positive PCR test of a culture analyzed for mycoplasma contamination, amplicon sequencing is still required for a final conclusion. However, the PCR test is approved by international expert organizations, and a sufficient number of kits for testing cell cultures for mycoplasma are available on the commercial market [28]. The primers used in commercial kits are ineffective for the detection of extracellular vesicles, but the discovery of specific sets of DNA nucleotide sequences in mycoplasma vesicles [29] opens up prospects for the development of PCR diagnostics for the detection of corresponding infectious agents.

In addition to PCR analysis for the detection of mycoplasmas, there are other methods—immunological and hybridization tests using antisera, monoclonal antibodies or DNA-RNA hybridization, involving the use of probes with a radioactive or fluorochrome label, as well as biochemical, microscopic and some other tests [30, 31].

These methods differ in sensitivity and are also not free from the disadvantages inherent in other methods for detecting mycoplasma contamination.

Thus, cultivating cell lines is a very labor-intensive process that requires cleanliness, attentiveness and professionalism of the working team.

5. The problems of malignant diseases and its treatment

There is a steady upward trend in new cases of cancer throughout the world. On the one hand, this is explained by more effective methods of early diagnosis, and on the other hand, by the aging of the population, environmental and economic reasons.

Mortality from cancer today is in second place after cardiovascular diseases, with a clear tendency to outstrip the latter. According to the World Health Organization, in 2022, there were an estimated 20 million new cancer cases and 9.7 million deaths, by 2030 the number of cancer cases reported annually worldwide will exceed 22.2 million. The estimated number of people who were alive within 5 years following a cancer diagnosis was 53.5 million. About 1 in 5 people develop cancer in their lifetime, approximately 1 in 9 men and 1 in 12 women die from the disease [32]. For long-term remission, timely and early diagnosis of the disease and properly selected therapy are extremely important.

A promising direction in cancer treatment is still the search for antitumor agents among plant objects. Currently, antitumor drugs used in the clinic contain *Vinca rosea* alkaloids—vinblastine, vincristine—as active components; *Taxus* sp. (taxanes)—paclitaxel, docetaxel; *Cólchicum speciósum*—colchamine, colchicine, as well as the podophyllotoxins etoposide and teniposide, isolated from *Podophyllum peltatum*. The antitumor effect of these alkaloids is due to their effect on cells in the M phase of the cell cycle (mitosis phase). Vinblastine and colchicine bind to microtubule tubulin molecules, due to their pronounced affinity, and prevent its polymerization, inhibit spindle formation (microtubule assembly) and stop mitosis at the metaphase stage [33]. Taxanes, on the contrary, increase the rate and degree of tubulin polymerization, stimulate the assembly of microtubules and prevent the depolymerization of this protein and the disintegration of microtubules. This process ultimately leads to disruption of the mitotic spindle formation process and inhibition of the cell cycle in G2 and M phases [34]. Widely used in clinical practice, etoposide and teniposide, according to their mechanism of action, are inhibitors of topoisomerases, enzymes involved in the process of DNA replication [35]. Despite advances in studying the causes and characteristics of cancer, as well as the availability of a huge number of chemotherapy drugs, including targeted ones, the incidence and mortality from cancer continue to increase. The fact is that the fundamental disadvantage of many chemotherapy drugs is their inability to selectively affect a malignant cell without affecting healthy cells of the body. Such "indiscrimination," as well as the mechanism of destruction of proliferating cells, lead to the high toxicity of chemotherapy. For example, treatment with vincristine in cancer patients with leukemia leads to nephrotoxicity due to its destabilization of microtubules of nervous tissue and subsequent activation of glycogen synthase kinase-3 [36]. Taxane causes muscle pain in patients with breast and lung cancer [37]. In connection with this, the relevance of further search for effective and safe cytostatics is only growing.

6. Isoquinolines and their derivatives as examples of the use of cellular models in *in vitro* cytotoxicity studies

Isoquinoline alkaloids occupy a special place among natural compounds, which is due to their structural diversity, high physiological activity and wide possibilities for obtaining biologically active substances based on them [38–41]. Simple isoquinolines have hemostatic activity, bis-benzylisoquinolines have analgesic [42], anti-inflammatory and anticonvulsant effects [43]. Among the 1,2,3,4-tetrahydroisoquinoline derivatives, compounds were found that exhibit the properties of central nervous system depressants [44], NMDA receptor blockers [45], antidiabetic activity [46]. There are also α-aminohydroxy-5-methyl-4-isoxazolepropionic acid (AMPA) receptor antagonists [47], selective orexin-2 receptor antagonists [48] and histamine H3 antagonists [49], compounds that cause bradycardia [50], as well as inhibitors of nitric oxide (NO) [51], serotonin uptake [49], γ-secretase [52] and vascular endothelial growth factor receptors (KDR) [53]. Literature data indicate high antibacterial activity of some tetrahydroisoquinolines. Thus, tetrahydroisoquinoline derivatives are highly selective against *Moraxella catarrhalis*, *Campylobacter jejuni* with MBC/MIC ≤4 [54], *Micobacter tuberculosis* [55], *S. pneumoniae* [56], as well as *Staphylococcus aureus* (MIC = 0.5 μg/ml), including a mecitillin-resistant strain [57]. Scientists from Boston's Northeastern University have synthesized a conjugate of the isoquinoline alkaloid berberine with a multidrug resistance inhibitor, which, being absolutely non-toxic to mammalian cells, exhibits high antimicrobial activity in a number of gram-positive bacteria with MIC = 1.8–3.7 μg/ml [57]. 2-Aryl-3,4-dihydroisoquinolin-2-iums were evaluated for antifungal activities *in vitro* against *Alternaria alternate*, *Curvularia lunata* and *Fusarium oxysporum sp. niveum* at 50 μg/ml. The structure–activity relationship indicated that the substituent in N-aromatic ring and its position had significant effect on the activity. The general trend was that halogen atoms and CF_3 remarkably enhanced the activity while CH_3 and OCH_3 decreased the activity. Generally, o-substituted isomers were more active than m- and p-substituted isomer [58].

Using *in vitro* methods, it was discovered that the target of tetrahydroisoquinolines in *M. tuberculosis* H37Rv was the ATP-dependent ligase MurE, a key enzyme involved in the early stage of cell wall peptidoglycan biosynthesis [55].

Several tetrahydroisoquinoline analogs containing lipid-like choline moiety were synthesized and evaluated for their antibacterial properties by Zablotskaya et al. [59]. These compounds also possessed inhibitory property against DNA gyrase, a vital enzyme that is involved in DNA topology.

FtsZ, a crucial protein in bacterial cell division has recently become of interest as target for the discovery of new antibacterial treatments. Tetrahydroisoquinoline ET770 showed antibacterial activities as shown by MIC and MBC values against *S. aureus* ATCC 25923, *Bacillus subtilis* ATCC 6633, MRSA DMST 20654, and *Escherichia coli* ATCC 25922. The elongation and filamentous forming of *E. coli* JW0093 cells were observed when treated with ET770 indicating the blockage of cell division process. It was indicated that tetrahydroisoquinoline ET770 had ability to inhibit bacterial FtsZ protein [60].

The wide range of biological activity of isoquinoline bases also includes antitumor properties. Thus, the macrolide isoquinoline alkaloids cyclepeltin, zephyranthine and methyltelobin-N have pronounced cytostatic activity and inhibit the growth of cervical carcinoma cells in low concentrations [61]. Isoquinoline 5-(2,6-difluorophenyl)-3-{[1-(methylsulfonyl)piperidin-4-yl]amino}-1H-pyrazolo[4,3-c]isoquinoline-7-carboxamide also showed a pronounced antitumor effect against these cancer cells with CE_{50} value 259 nM.

Various derivatives have also proven effective against breast cancer [62]. 3N-(4-methylbenzoyl) and 3K-(4-methoxybenzoyl)–derivatives of 3-benzoylamino-6,7-dimethoxy-1-methylisoquinoline are known in the literature, which exhibit high cytotoxic activity against CaOV ovarian carcinoma cells. The tetrahydroisoquinoline alkaloid renieramycin M, isolated from the blue sponge *Xestospongia* sp., is active against H460 lung cancer cells. This alkaloid shows high cytotoxicity and antimetastatic activity with an IC_{50} value of 40 μM [63]. Tetrahydroisoquinolines are also active against glioblastoma, the most aggressive form of brain tumor, and carcinomas. The substance EDL-360 (12) serves as a powerful antiglioma agent against the LN18 cell line (IC_{50}: 5.42 ± 0.06 μM), in which the functional group is the carbon linker between the biphenyl and the tetrahydroisoquinoline ring [64]. Japanese scientists, studying the tumor specificity of 1,2,3,4-tetrahydroisoquinolines on oral carcinoma cell lines, showed that the presence of a 3,4-dimethoxybenzoyl group at position C-2 (R3), an ethoxycarbonyl substituent at C-1 (R2) and benzyloxycarbonyl radical at C-2 (R3) leads to the highest cytotoxicity and tumor specificity of the compounds [65]. The results obtained confirm earlier studies by another Japanese scientific group, where it was established that the presence of alkyl substituents 1-cyclobutyl-, 1-cyclohexyl-, 1-phenyl or 1-benzylate at the C-1 position of the isoquinoline molecule causes significant death of pheochromocytoma of the adrenal medulla PC12 by triggering apoptosis [66]. It is interesting to note that in the literature there is information about tetrahydroichoisoquinolines that overcome multidrug resistance of tumor cells [67, 68]. The experimental antitumor drug Pixantrone (Cell Therapeutics, USA), marketed under the brand name Pixuvri, contains the isoquinoline derivative 6,9-bis(2-aminoethylamino)benzoisoquinoline-5,10-dione as an active base. The mechanism of cytotoxic action of pixantrone is inhibition of topoisomerase II and DNA intercalation. The cytotoxicity of the drug is not accompanied by oxidative stress [69]. A distinctive feature of this antitumor agent is its slight toxic effect on heart tissue.

Often, semi-industrial production of biologically active substances from natural sources of plant or other origin is difficult due to the difficulty of purifying them from impurities or due to their low content. In such cases, the attention of researchers is drawn to the synthetic preparation of both the compound itself and its chemical modification aimed at enhancing physiological activity and (or) reducing side effects. Tetrahydroisoquinolines, whose molecules have one or more reaction centers, contain wide synthetic possibilities and therefore have long attracted the attention of specialists in the field of organic chemistry.

Thus, in a number of experiments, the *in vitro* cytotoxicity of three types of tetrahydroisoquinoline was studied: monoderivatives - synthetic derivatives of the alkaloids cryptostyline and salsolidine, bimolecular tetrahydroisoquinolines-1,4-bis(6,7-dimethoxy- and 1,4-bis(6,7-methylenedioxy-1,2,3,4-tetrahydroisoquinolin-1-yl) alkanes and conjugates of isoquinolines and the bioflavonoid dihydroquercetin (DHQ) [70, 71]. It has been established that the chemical cross-linking of alkaloids and amines with dihydroquercetin entails the complete disappearance of the cytotoxic properties of the substances, and in some cases leads to high proliferative activity of cancer cells. At the same time, it was found that the synergistic effect of individual components does not cause either proliferation or suppression of the growth of cancer cells, in contrast to their synthetic complexes. As it turned out, the necessary conditions for the manifestation of cytotoxicity in monoderivatives are the presence of 2 methoxy substituents in ring A, a free N atom, as well as the presence of a benzene ring with methylenedioxy groups and halogens or a hydrophobic group at the C-1 position of tetrahydroisoquinoline. Moreover, the amount of $(-CH_2-)$ at the C-1 position of the molecule is also a critical indicator for cytotoxicity. So, if the IC_{50} value for sample $(-CH_2-)_7$ was 32–42 μM on the CCRF-CEM, HEp-2, HBL-100, HeLa lines, then for tetrahydroisoquinoline $(-CH_2-)_{13}$ this value was 3–10.2 μM at SI > 5. As for 1,4-bis(6,7-dimethoxy- and 1,4-bis(6,7-methylenedioxy-1,2,3,4-tetrahydroisoquinolin-1-yl) alkanes, it was found that the introduction into the isoquinoline structure of the second molecule retained the high cytostatic effect of the substance and reduced selectivity to cancer cell lines [71]. It was determined that the sequential addition of $-CH_2-$ groups between tetrahydroisoquinoline molecules increases both the

DOI: http://dx.doi.org/10.5772/intechopen.1008310

percentage of suppression of cell growth and reduces the specificity of substances to cell lines. Thus, the greatest cytotoxic effect was demonstrated by bimolecular tetrahydroisoquinolines with $(-CH_2-)_8$ and $(-CH_2-)_{11}$, showing an IC_{50} value of 2–4 μM and SI > 8.

Studying the mechanism of cytotoxicity of these tetrahydroisoquinolines showed that the derivatives caused apoptosis in cancer cells by reducing the activity of the Bcl-2 gene and activating the Bax gene, as well as activation of caspases 3 and 7. At the same time, the cytotoxicity of isoquinolines with a hydrophobic group at the C-1 position was accompanied by oxidative stress, but only in cancer cells, and in healthy cells these compounds showed antioxidant effects. It is interesting to note that among monoderivatives with the presence of methylenedioxy groups and halogens, 1,4-bis(6,7-dimethoxy- and 1,4-bis(6,7-methylenedioxy-1,2,3,4-tetrahydroisoquinoline-1-yl)alkanes and synthetic conjugates of isoquinolines and the bioflavonoid DHQ, cytotoxicity was not accompanied by oxidative stress.

It has been revealed that most isoquinoline compounds affect the DNA repair of cancer cells [72, 73]. Thus, the authors present a wide range of isoquinolines and dihydroisoquinolines that inhibit polyadenosine diphosphoribose polymerase—PARP [74]. Suppression of the activity of this enzyme leads to the lethal outcome of a number of cancer cells defective in the repair of double-strand DNA breaks, which depends on homologous recombination and inhibitors of tubulin polymerization [75]. Mitogen-activated protein kinases ERK1/2 and MEK1 were identified as molecular targets of some tetrahydroisoquinolines in mediating NSCLC apoptosis [76]. CDKs (cyclin-dependent kinases) are serine/threonine kinases enzymes that play a crucial role in regulating eukaryotic cell cycle, apoptosis, differentiation, and transcription. The enzyme dihydrofolate reductase (DHFR) catalyzes the reduction of dihydrofolate to tetrahydrofolate, essential for DNA synthesis, cell growth, and the production of raw materials for cell proliferation in cancer cells. So, 5,6,7,8-(tetrahydroisoquinolin 3-yl)thio compounds and related 6,7,8,9-tetrahyrothieno[2,3-c]isoquinolines incorporating 4-(N,N-dimethylamino) phenyl moiety showed significant inhibition of CDK2 and DHFR enzymes [77].

Recent evidence has suggested that the poor response to the current treatment drugs and the ability to undergo metastasis are driven by cancer stem cells (CSCs) within the tumor. 5-O-acetyl-renieramycin T (marine tetrahydroisoquinoline derivative) isolated from the blue sponge *Xestospongia* sp. mediated lung cancer cell death via the induction of p53-dependent apoptosis and induced the death of CSCs as represented by the CSC markers CD44 and CD133, while the stem cell transcription factor Nanog was also found to be dramatically decreased in 5-O-acetyl-renieramycin T-treated cells. CSC suppression was due to the ability of the compound to deplete the protein kinase B (AKT) signal [78].

7. Conclusion

Thus, *in vitro* cell models make it possible to conduct full tests of biologically active substances, study their different biological effects, identify the mechanisms of their action, and select the most promising samples for future *in vivo* studies.

Author details

Terenteva Ekaterina Olegovna[1*], Khashimova Zaynat Sattarovna[2], Khamidova Umida Bakhriddin Kizi[1], Umarova Mukaddas Rustamovna[1], Tosheva Nigora Arziyevna[1], Alimukhamedova Orzigul Bakhrievna[1] and Azimova Shakhnoz Sadikovna[1]

1 The Institute of the Chemistry of Plant Substances named after Acad. S.Yu.Yunusov, Republic of Uzbekistan

2 Academy of Sciences of Uzbekistan, Institute of Bioorganic Chemistry, Republic of Uzbekistan

*Address all correspondence to: terenteva_katerina@bk.ru

References

[1] Eskov AP. Toxicological tests: Alternative methods. Toxicological Bulletin. 2003;**5**:25-29

[2] Blazhevich OV. Cell Cultivation: Course of Lectures. Minsk: BSU; 2004. p. 50. (In Russian)

[3] Epstein RJ. A periodic table for cancer. Future Oncology. 2015;**11**(5):785-800

[4] Baraboy VA, Brekhman II, Golozhin VG. Peroxidation and Stress. Moscow: Science; 2004. p. 148. (In Russian)

[5] Eropkin MY, Smirnova TD, Eropkina EM, et al. Study of the participation of calcium ions in the toxic effect of xenobiotics on human cells in culture. Cytology. 2000;**42**(2):154-159. (In Russian)

[6] Gillet JP, Varma S, Gottesman MM. The clinical relevance of cancer cell lines. Journal of the National Cancer Institute. 2013;**105**(7):452-458. DOI: 10.1093/jnci/djt007

[7] Jia L, Lin H, Oppenheim J, Zack Howard OM, Li J, Fan H, et al. US National Cancer Institute–China collaborative studies on Chinese medicine and cancer. JNCI Monographs. 2017;**2017**(52):lgx007. DOI: 10.1093/jncimonographs/lgx007

[8] OECD Principles on Good Laboratory Practice, ENV/MC/CHEM(98)17. 1997. pp. 22-28

[9] Melnikova NA, Shubina OS, Dudenkova NA, Lapshina MV, Liferenko OV, Timoshkina OI. Study of cell viability under the influence of lead acetate on the rat body: Modern problems of science and education. 2013;**5**. (In Russian). Available from: https://science-education.ru/ru/article/view?id=10588

[10] Repetto G, del Peso A, Zurita JL. Neutral red uptake assay for the estimation of cell viability/cytotoxicity. Nature Protocols. 2008;**3**(7):1125-1131. DOI: 10.1038/nprot.2008

[11] Ghasemi M, Turnbull T, Sebastian S, Kempson I. The MTT assay: Utility, limitations, pitfalls, and interpretation in bulk and single-cell analysis. International Journal of Molecular Sciences. 2021;**22**(23):12827. DOI: 10.3390/ijms222312827

[12] Vichai V, Kirtikara K. Sulforhodamine B colorimetric assay for cytotoxicity screening. Nature Protocols. 2006;**1**:1112-1116

[13] Kaja S, Payne AJ, Naumchuk Y, Koulen P. Quantification of lactate dehydrogenase for cell viability testing using cell lines and primary cultured astrocytes. Current Protocols in Toxicology. 2017;**72**:2.26.1-2.26.10. DOI: 10.1002/cptx.21

[14] Protocol for the EZ4U Cell Proliferation and Cytotoxicity Assay kit, Biomedica CAT. NO. BI-5000 10 X 96 DETEREMINATIONS. Biomedica rev.no. 190104 (replacing 160725)

[15] Belikova AM, Zarytova VF, Grineva NI. Synthesis of ribonucleosides and diribonucleoside phosphates containing 2-chloro-ethylamine and nitrogen mustard residues. Tetrahedron Letters. 1967;**37**:3557-3562

[16] Grineva NI, Karpova GG. Complementarily targeted alkylation of ribosomal RNA by alkylating

oligonucleotide derivatives. Molecular Biology. 1974;**8**:832-844. (In Russian)

[17] Grineva NI, Karpova GG, Kuznetsova LM, Uimitova TA, Venksternl TB. Complementarily addressed alkylation of yeast tRNA 1 Val with chloroethylmethyl-aminobenzylidene d(pC-G)-A. Proof of the modification of the third nucleotide located at the 5'-terminus of the complete binding site of the reagent. Molecular Biology. 1976;**10**:1260-1271. (In Russian)

[18] Zamecnik PC, Stephenson ML. Inhibition of Rous sarcoma virus replication and cell transformation by a specific oligodeoxynucleotide. Proceedings of the National Academy ofSciences of the United States of America. 1978;**75**(1):280-284

[19] Falvey AK, Kantor JA, Robert-Guroff MG, Picciano DJ, Weiss GB, Vavich JM, et al. Mechanism of Action of Ribonucleic Acid-directed Deoxyribonucleic Acid Polymerase: I. Transcription of globin messenger ribonucleic acid. The Journal of Biological Chemistry. 1974;**249**(22):7049-7056

[20] Uphoff C, Drexler H. Elimination of mycoplasmas from infected cell lines using antibiotics. Methods in Molecular Biology. 2011;**731**:105114

[21] Rottem S, Kosower N, Kornspan JD. Contamination of Tissue Cultures by Mycoplasmas. Biology, Medicine. IntechOpen Science. Chapter 3. 2012. pp. 35-58

[22] Borkhsenius SN, Chernova OA, Chernov VM, Vonsky MS. Mycoplasmas. St. Petersburg: Nauka; 2002. p. 320. (In Russian)

[23] Chernov VM, Chernova OA, Sanchez-Vega HT, Kolpakov AI, Ilyinskaya ON. Mycoplasma contamination of cell cultures: Vesicular traffic in bacteria and the problem of controlling infectious agents. Actanaturae. 2014;**6**:43-54. (In Russian)

[24] Drexler HG, Uphoff CC. Mycoplasma contamination of cell cultures: Incidence, sources, effects, detection, elimination, prevention. Cytotechnology. 2002;**39**(2):75-90

[25] Rottem S. Interaction of mycoplasmas with host cells. Physiological Reviews. 2003;**83**(2):417-432

[26] Harasawa R, Mizusawa H, Fujii M, Yamamoto J, Mukai H, Uemori T, et al. Rapid detection and differentiation of the major mycoplasma contaminants in cell cultures using real-time PCR with SYBR Green I and melting curve analysis. Microbiology and Immunology. 2005;**49**(9):859-863

[27] Sung H, Kang SH, Bae YJ, Hong JT, Chung YB, Lee CK, et al. PCR-based detection of mycoplasma species. Journal of Microbiology. 2006;**44**(1):42-49

[28] Uphoff CC, Drexler HG. Detection of mycoplasma contaminations. Methods in Molecular Biology. 2013;**946**:1-13

[29] Chernov VM, Chernova OA, Mouzykantov AA, Baranova NB, Gorshkov OV, Trushin MV, et al. Extracellular membrane vesicles and phytopathogenicity of *Acholeplasmalaidlawii* PG8. Scientific World Journal. 2012;**2012**:Article 315474. DOI: 10.1100/2012/315474

[30] Mariotti E, D'Alessio F, Mirabelli P, Di Noto R, Fortunato G, Del Vecchio L. *Mollicutes* contamination: A new strategy for an effective rescue of cancer cell lines. Biologicals. 2012;**40**(1):88-91

[31] Degeling MH, Maguire CA, Bovenberg MS, Tannous BA. Sensitive

assay for mycoplasma detection in mammalian cell culture. Analytical Chemistry. 2012;**84**(9):4227-4232

[32] World Health Organization. Available from: https://www.who.int/news/item/01-02-2024-global-cancerburden-growing--amidst-mountingneed-for-services

[33] Lu Y, Chen J, Xiao M, Li W, Miller DD. An overview of tubulin inhibitors that interact with the colchicine binding site. Pharmaceutical Research. 2012;**29**(11):2943-2971. DOI: 10.1007/s11095-012-0828-z

[34] Fu Y, Li S, Zu Y, Yang G, Yang Z, Luo M, et al. Medicinal chemistry of paclitaxel and its analogues. Current Medicinal Chemistry. 2009;**16**(30):3966-3985

[35] Nitiss JL. Targeting DNA topoisomerase II in cancer chemotherapy. Nature Reviews Cancer. 2009;**9**(5):338-350

[36] Alimoradi H, Pourmohammadi N, Mehr SE, et al. Effects of lithium on peripheral neuropathy induced by vincristine in rats. Acta Medica Iranica. 2012;**50**:373-379

[37] Heney M, Alipour M, Vergidis D, Omri A, Mugabe C, Th'ng J, et al. Effectiveness of liposomal paclitaxel against MCF-7 breast cancer cells. Canadian Journal of Physiology and Pharmacology. 2010;**88**:1172-1180

[38] Chen C, Wu J, Zhu P, Xu C, Yao L. Investigating isoquinoline derivatives for inhibition of inhibitor of apoptosis proteins for ovarian cancer treatment. Drug Design, Development and Therapy. 2017;**11**:2697-2707

[39] Dembitsky VM, Gloriozova TA, Poroikov VV. Naturally occurring plant isoquinoline N-oxide alkaloids: Their pharmacological and SAR activities. Phytomedicine. 2015;**22**(1):183-202

[40] Mihoubi M, Micale N, Scala A, Jarraya RM, Bouaziz A, et al. Synthesis of C3/C1-substituted tetrahydroisoquinolines. Molecules. 2015;**20**(8):14902-14914

[41] Zablotskaya A, Segal I, Geronikaki A, Eremkina T, Belyakov S, et al. Synthesis, physicochemical characterization, cytotoxicity, antimicrobial, antiinflammatory and psychotropic activity of new N-[1,3-(benzo)thiazol-2-yl]- ω-[3,4-dihydroisoquinolin-2(1H)-yl] alkanamides. European Journal of Medicinal Chemistry. 2013;**70**:846-856. DOI: 10.1016/j.ejmech.2013.10.008

[42] Tursunkhojaeva FM, Rakhimov SB, Dzhahangirov FN, Vinogradova VI, Rezhepov Z, Sagdullaev SS. 1-(4′-Methoxyphenyl)-2β-Hydroxyethyl6,7-Dimethoxy-1,2,3,4-Tetrahydroichoquinoline Hydrochloride (1), Exhibiting Local Anesthetic and Analgesic Effects [Patent Uz IAP 04590; IAP 2010 0136]. 2012

[43] Shamma M, Moniot JL. The Isoquinoline Alkaloids Research 1972-1977. New York: C.X. Maex; 1978. pp. 84-88

[44] Ott H, Hardtmann GE, Denzer M, Frey AJ, Gogerty JH, Leslie GH, et al. Tetrahydroisoquino[2,1-d][1,4] benzodiazepines: Synthesis and neuropharmacological activity. Journal of Medicinal Chemistry. 1968;**11**(4):777-787. DOI: 10.1021/jm00310a610

[45] Wanner KT, Beer H, Höfner G, Ludwig M. Asymmetric synthesis and enantioselectivity of binding of 1-aryl-1,2,3,4-tetrahydroisoquinolines at the PCP site of the NMDA-receptor complex.

European Journal of Organic Chemistry. 1998;**9**:2019-2029

[46] Azukizawa S, Kasai M, Takahashi K, Mike T, Kunishiro K, Kanda M, et al. Synthesis and biological evaluation of (S)-1,2,3,4-tetrahydroisoquinoline-3-carboxylic acids: A novel series of PPARγ agonists. Chemical & Pharmaceutical Bulletin. 2008;**56**:335-345

[47] Gitto R, Ficarra R, Stancanelli R, Guardo M, De Luca L, Barreca ML, et al. Synthesis, resolution, stereochemistry, and molecular modeling of (R)- and (S)-2-acetyl-1-(4′-chlorophenyl)-6,7-dimethoxy-1,2,3,4-tetrahydroisoquinoline AMPAR antagonists. Bioorganic & Medicinal Chemistry. 2007;**15**:5417-5423

[48] Hirose M, Egashira S, Goto Y, Hashihayata T, Ohtake N, Iwaasa H, et al. N-Acyl 6,7-dimethoxy-1,2,3,4-tetrahydroisoquinoline: The first orexin-2 receptor selective non-peptidic antagonist. Bioorganic & Medicinal Chemistry Letters. 2003;**13**:4497-4499

[49] Letavic MA, Keith JM, Jablonowski JA, Stocking EM, Gomez LA, Ly KS, et al. Novel tetrahydroisoquinolines are histamine H3 antagonists and serotonin reuptake inhibitors. Bioorganic & Medicinal Chemistry Letters. 2007;**17**:1047-1051

[50] Kubota H, Watanabe T, Kakefuda A, Masuda N, Wada K, Ishii N, et al. Synthesis and pharmacological evaluation of piperidinoalkanoyl-1,2,3,4-tetrahydroisoquinoline derivatives as novel specific bradycardic agents. Bioorganic & Medicinal Chemistry Letters. 2004;**14**:3049-3052

[51] Seo JW, Srisook E, Son HJ, Hwang O, Cha YN, Chi DY. Synthesis of tetrahydroisoquinoline derivatives that inhibit NO production in activated BV-2 microglial cells. European Journal of Medicinal Chemistry. 2008;**43**:1160-1170

[52] Hu MK, Liao YF, Chen JF, Wang BJ, Tung YT, Lin HC, et al. New 1,2,3,4-tetrahydroisoquinoline derivatives as modulators of proteolytic cleavage of amyloid precursor proteins. Bioorganic & Medicinal Chemistry. 2008;**16**:1957-1965

[53] Choquette D, Teffera Y, Polverino A, Harmange JC. Discovery of novel 1,2,3,4-tetrahydroisoquinolines and 3,4-dihydroisoquinoline-1(2H)-ones as potent and selective inhibitors of KDR: Synthesis, SAR, and pharmacokinetic properties. Bioorganic & Medicinal Chemistry Letters. 2008;**18**:4054-4058

[54] Bielawski K, Leszczyńska K, Kałuża Z, Bielawska A, Michalak O, Daniluk T, et al. Synthesis and antimicrobial activity of chiral quaternary N-spiro ammonium bromides with 3′,4′-dihydro-1'H-spiro[isoindoline-2,2′-isoquinoline] skeleton. Drug Design, Development and Therapy. 2017;**11**:2015-2028. DOI: 10.2147/DDDT.S133250

[55] Guzman JD, Pesnot T, Barrera DA, Davies HM, McMahon E, Evangelopoulos D, et al. Tetrahydroisoquinolines affect the whole-cell phenotype of *Mycobacterium tuberculosis* by inhibiting the ATP-dependent MurE ligase. Journal of Antimicrobial Chemotherapy. 2015;**70**(6):1691-1703. DOI: 10.1093/jac/dkv010

[56] Panchaud P, Bruyère T, Blumstein AC, Bur D, Chambovey A, Ertel EA, et al. Discovery and optimization of isoquinoline ethyl ureas as antibacterial agents. Journal of Medicinal Chemistry. 2017;**60**(9):3755-3775. DOI: 10.1021/acs.jmedchem.6b01834

[57] Cushnie TP, Cushnie BT, Lamb AJ. Alkaloids: An overview of their antibacterial, antibiotic-enhancing and antivirulence activities. International Journal of Antimicrobial Agents. 2014;**44**:377-386

[58] Yang X, Yao Y, Qin Y, Hou Z, Yang R, Miao F, et al. Synthesis and in vitro antifungal activities of new 2-aryl-6,7-methylenedioxy-3,4-dihydroisoquinolin-2-ium bromides. Chemical and Pharmaceutical Bulletin. 2013;**61**(7):731-739. DOI: 10.1248/cpb.c13-00221

[59] Zablotskaya A, Segal I, Geronikaki A, Shestakova I, Nikolajeva V, Makarenkova G. N-Heterocyclic choline analogues based on 1,2,3,4-tetrahydro (iso)quinoline scaffold with anticancer and anti-infective dual action. Pharmacological Reports. 2017;**69**:575-581. DOI: 10.1016/j.pharep.2017.01.028

[60] Charoenwiwattanakij P, Pratuangdejkul J, Jaturanpinyo M, Lowtangkitcharoen W, Suwanborirux K, Nukoolkarn V. Ecteinascidin 770, a tetrahydroisoquinoline alkaloid, targeting the bacterial cell division protein FtsZ. Chiang Mai Journal of Science. 2018;**45**(7):2566-2580

[61] Kartsev VG, Tolstikova GA. Nitrogen Heterocycles and Alkaloids. Moscow; 2001. pp. 97-98

[62] Lin HR, Safo MK, Abraham DJ. Identification of a series of tetrahydroisoquinoline derivatives as potential therapeutic agents for breast cancer. Bioorganic & Medicinal Chemistry Letters. 2007;**17**(9):2581-2589. DOI: 10.1016/j.bmcl.2007.02.002

[63] Halim H, Chunhacha P, Suwanborirux K, Chanvorachote P. Anticancer and antimetastatic activities of Renieramycin M, a marine tetrahydroisoquinoline alkaloid, in human non-small cell lung cancer cells. Anticancer Research. 2011;**31**(1):193-201

[64] Patil R, Hosni-Ahmed A, Jones TS, Patil SA, Asres LB, Wang X, et al. Synthesis and in vitro evaluation of novel 1,2,3,4-tetrahydroisoquinoline derivatives as potent antiglioma agents. Anti-Cancer Agents in Medicinal Chemistry. 2014;**14**(3):473-482

[65] Hatano H, Takekawa F, Hashimoto K, Ishihara M, Kawase M, Qing C, et al. Tumor-specific cytotoxic activity of 1,2,3,4-tetrahydroisoquinoline derivatives against human oral squamous cell carcinoma cell lines. Anticancer Research. 2009;**29**:3079-3086

[66] Saitoh T, Abe K, Ishikawa M, Nakatani M, Shimazu S, Satoh N, et al. Synthesis and in vitro cytotoxicity of 1,2,3,4-tetrahydroisoquinoline derivatives. European Journal of Medicinal Chemistry. 2006;**41**:241-253

[67] Yan F, Jiang Y, Li Y-M, Zhen X, Cen J, Fang W-R. Reversal of P-glycoprotein and multidrug resistance-associated protein 1-mediated multidrug resistance in cancer cells by HZ08 isomers, tetraisohydroquinoline derivatives. Biological & Pharmaceutical Bulletin. 2008;**31**:1258-1264

[68] Li Y, Zhang HB, Huang WL, Li YM. Design and synthesis of tetrahydroisoquinoline derivatives as potential multidrug resistance reversal agents in cancer. Bioorganic & Medicinal Chemistry Letters. 2008;**18**:3652-3655

[69] Lekue BC, Cicala GS, Leppä S, et al. Pixantrone beyond monotherapy: A review. Annals of Hematology. 2019;**98**:2025-2033. DOI: 10.1007/s00277-019-03749-0

[70] Terent′eva EO, Saidov AS, Khashimova ZS, Tseomashko NE, Sasmakov SA, Abdurakhmanov DM, et al. Synthesis and biological activity of 1,11-bis(6,7-methylenedioxyand 6,7-dimethoxy-1,2,3,4-tetrahydroisoquinolin-1-yl)undecanes. Chemistry of Natural Compounds. 2017;**53**(2):328-332

[71] Terenteva EO, Khashimova ZS, Tsay EA, Zhurakulov SN, Saidov AS, Vinogradova VI, et al. Chemical modification of tetrahydroisoquinolines and their cytotoxic activity. Asian Journal of Pharmacy and Pharmacology. 2017;**3**(3):66-78

[72] Phenanthridinone as Poly (ADP-Ribose) Polymerase Inhibitors [EP Patent No. 1487800]. Kouji c/o Fujisawa Pharm. Co. Ltd HATTORI, Koichiro c/o Fujisawa Pharm. Co. Ltd MUKOYOSHI, Hirofumi c/o Fujisawa Pharm. Co. Ltd YAMAMOTO; 2004

[73] Mabire DJ, Guillemont JE, Van Dun JAJ, Somers MVF, Wouters WBL. 7-Phenylalkyl Substituted 2-Quinolinones and 2-Quinoxalinones as Poly(ADP-Ribose) Polymerase Inhibitors [EP Patent No. 1709011]. 2005

[74] Pellicciari R, Moroni F. Thieno[2,3-c] isoquinolines for use as inhibitors of PARP [US Patent No 0094746A1]. 2006

[75] Xu L, Huang G, Zhu Z, Tian S, Wei Y, Hong H, et al. LFZ-4-46, a tetrahydroisoquinoline derivative, induces apoptosis and cell cycle arrest via induction of DNA damage and activation of MAPKs pathway in cancer cells. Anti-Cancer Drugs. 2021;**32**(8):842-854. DOI: 10.1097/CAD.0000000000001077

[76] Iksen I, Sinsook S, Wattanathamsan O, Buaban K, Chamni S, Pongrakhananon V. Target identification of 22-(4-pyridinecarbonyl) jorunnamycin A, a tetrahydroisoquinoline derivative from the sponge *Xestospongia* sp., in mediating non-small-cell lung cancer cell apoptosis. Molecules. 2022;**27**(24):8948. DOI: 10.3390/molecules27248948

[77] Sayed EM, Bakhite EA, Hassanien R, Farhan N, Aly HF, Morsy SG, et al. Novel tetrahydroisoquinolines as DHFR and CDK2 inhibitors: Synthesis, characterization, anticancer activity and antioxidant properties. BMC Chemistry. 2024;**18** Article number: 34

[78] Chantarawong W, Chamni S, Suwanborirux K, Saito N, Chanvorachote P. 5-*O*-Acetyl-renieramycin T from blue sponge *Xestospongia* sp. induces lung cancer stem cell apoptosis. Marine Drugs. 2019;**17**(2):109. DOI: 10.3390/md17020109

Chapter 6

Addressing Challenges in Cell Lysis: Effective Strategies and Technologies

Pragya Prakash, Shoaib Haidar and Hare Ram Singh

Abstract

Cell lysis and disruption involve breaking down cells through natural processes or induced damage to the outer membrane. This process can occur during apoptosis, which helps detoxify and clear cells. However, when extracting valuable intracellular products from microbial or mammalian cells, controlled lysis techniques are essential. Lysis and cytotoxicity can lead to loss of desired products, toxin production, and complications from exopolysaccharides and endotoxins. While it may aid in detoxification when regulated, uncontrolled cytotoxicity complicates product extraction. To address these issues, researchers are developing novel extraction strategies tailored to the type of cells and the stability of the target products. Methods for cell disruption include physical, biological, and chemical approaches, with physical techniques often favoured in biological applications to enhance product recovery. The current chapter will provide an insight into the recent developments in the field of cell disruption, analysis of cell toxicity, and challenges associated with the phenomena. This chapter explores the various obstacles encountered in the process of cell lysis, a critical step in bioprocessing. This chapter delves into the underlying principles of cell lysis, examines the most common issues faced by researchers, and presents innovative strategies and cutting-edge technologies designed to overcome these challenges.

Keywords: cell lysis, cell disruption, cytotoxicity, intracellular products, exopolysaccharides

1. Introduction

Cell lysis and cell disruption refer to the breakdown of cells by self-induction or induced damage to the outer membrane. The cell lysis is carried out under various conditions, and with time multiple techniques have been developed for cell disruption. Naturally, cell lysis occurs with the cells entering apoptosis whenever there is a need for detoxification and clearance of cells. However, since a number of biological products are being produced using microbial or mammalian cells, cell lysis is performed to get the intracellular product in its crude form [1]. There are numerous challenges researchers face when moving with lysis methods and one of them is

IntechOpen

cytotoxicity. Cytotoxicity is the effect of internal or external stimuli/environment leading to cell death [2]. The result of cytotoxicity is loss of product, production of toxins, and availability of exopolysaccharides and endotoxins. The cytotoxicity leads to multiple complications because of cellular material on availability and stability of the desired product. While cytotoxicity leads to clearance of toxins and when in controlled form is good as a natural maintenance of cellular systems, its induction and uncontrolled nature may lead to serious complications while extracting a desired product [3].

Cytotoxicity is one issue related to cell lysis while the procedures performed for inducing cell lysis also creates many barriers to the extraction of the desired product. With the development of novel strategies for the extraction of intracellular products, the focus has been to develop strategies keeping in mind the recovery of the desired product. Depending on the type and class of cells and the sensitivity, and stability of the material, the strategy is decided. It can be physical methods, biological, and chemical methods. In terms of biological applications, the physical methods for cell disruption are usually used [4].

2. What is cytotoxicity?

2.1 Cytotoxicity and its prediction

Cytotoxicity refers to the quality of being toxic to cells, which can result from various factors, including chemical exposure, radiation, and biological agents. The chapter highlights the significance of studying cytotoxicity, particularly in the context of cancer treatment and environmental toxicology. Understanding how different substances affect cell viability is crucial for developing effective therapeutic strategies and assessing the safety of chemicals [5].

Cytotoxicity is the adverse effects observed from reactions with internal or external factors such as metal ions, chemicals, phytotoxins or microbial infections. Once the cytotoxicity is observed the immune system responds to it by inducing apoptosis and clearance from the system. Depending upon how the cells are impulsive for cytotoxic agents, it results in a variety of prognoses. While it may induce apoptosis, i.e., programmed cell death, it may also induce necrosis, and as a result, cell may undergo lysis. As cytotoxicity is important in biological and specifically physiological processes, it becomes important to measure the cytotoxicity to determine its extent and further plan its control if needed. Cytotoxicity is measured in multiple ways and one of the common strategies is ATP measurement. The basic mechanism behind the estimation of cytotoxicity is that, due to altered cellular membranes, the cellular material leaks out of the cell and hence allows space for the labeling dyes to penetrate through. This mechanism of uptake of dyes by cells, however, can lead to inaccurate estimation of cytotoxicity. To overcome this, modern non-radiolabeled methods have been developed which act on the specific class of molecules present in both proliferating and non-proliferating cells to determine cytotoxicity.

2.2 Analysis of cytotoxicity

The analysis of cytotoxicity can be divided into several types. Some are traditional, while others are newly developed and focus on the evolving needs of the future.

DOI: http://dx.doi.org/10.5772/intechopen.1008313

2.2.1 Agar overlay test

The agar overlay test is a traditionally used method to determine the toxic effects of various materials on living cells. It is used to test toxicity toward bacterial cells or any particular bacterial strain. This involves careful preparation of an extract or purified material to be tested for cytotoxicity, as the purity of the material and external environmental conditions may lead to false results. Also, this method cannot be used to determine cytotoxicity in animal cell culture and hence has limited applications [6].

2.2.2 MTT assay

The MTT assay is the most common assay to study cytotoxicity in animal cell culture. The MTT reagent (3-(4,5-dimethylthiazol-2-yl)-2,5-diphenyl-2H-tetrazolium bromide) is a mono-tetrazolium salt that consists of a positively charged quaternary tetrazole ring core containing four nitrogen atoms surrounded by three aromatic rings including two phenyl moieties and one thiazolyl ring. The reaction leads to the reduction of MTT which results in disruption of the core tetrazole ring and the formation of a violet-blue water-insoluble molecule called formazan. The MTT assay has multiple applications in cancer research and drug development. It also helps in the development of new cell lines and is also used for the analysis of stable cell lines. Adapting to modern-day research this can also be used for high-throughput screening applications [7].

Despite the applications, this method has many limitations, and various factors contribute to its misinterpretation of results. One of the limitations is that the measurement of cellular toxicity is based on the metabolic activity and not on cell viability, which may lead to false interpretation as the low metabolic activity cell may be viable. Also, the non-viable cells can be metabolically active for some or longer duration of time [7]. Like the agar test the MTT test is also impacted by environmental factors such as temperature, pH, osmolarity, and other than that cell density.

Since the MTT assay is not always automated, hence, there are high chances of manual errors while handling the cell lines, storage and preparation of reagents, delay time, and mechanical errors. While these errors are tough to avoid, one of the common errors that happens is the designing of experiments and protocols. It is important to note here that for every cell line or treatment condition, the MTT assay protocol changes, and hence, it is difficult to avoid inaccuracy at certain levels. However, despite the limitations and vulnerability, MTT assay remains a popular test of cytotoxicity due to its replicability, ease of doing, and cost-effectiveness [8]. However, it is needed to put in controls so that the impact of external factors can be minimized. Also, the automation of the MTT assay could lead to a reduction in manual and mechanical errors.

2.2.3 Cytokinesis-block micronucleus-cytome assay

This is a comprehensive method which measures cytotoxicity based on DNA damage. Multiple events such as binucleated cells, presence of micronuclei, chromosome loss, and chromosome damage are counted as scores. A ratio of binucleated and multinucleated cells to the necrotic and/or apoptotic cells is taken into consideration. More information on the DNA damage is sought using centromere or telomere probes. The assay is applied for analysis of in-vivo genotoxin exposure and *in-vitro* genotoxicity test [9].

2.2.3.1 Methodology

1. Sample preparation: Whole blood is diluted and layered over Ficoll-Paque to separate leukocytes. After centrifugation, the leukocyte layer is collected and further processed to obtain a pure lymphocyte suspension.

2. Cell culture: The isolated lymphocytes are cultured in a suitable medium, typically supplemented with fetal bovine serum (FBS). The article corrects a previous error regarding the concentration of FBS required, emphasizing the need for a 100% solution.

3. Cytokinesis block: A key feature of the assay is the use of cytochalasin B, which inhibits cytokinesis, allowing for the formation of binucleated cells. This step is crucial for the accurate scoring of micronuclei.

4. Slide preparation: The article details the process of cytocentrifugation to prepare slides for microscopic examination. Proper slide preparation is critical for obtaining clear and interpretable results.

5. Staining and scoring: After air-drying and fixing the slides, cells are stained to visualize the micronuclei. The scoring of micronuclei is performed under a microscope, where the number of micronuclei per 1000 binucleated cells is counted. The article emphasizes the importance of maintaining consistent scoring criteria to ensure reproducibility.

2.2.3.2 Applications of the CBMN assay

The CBMN assay has a wide range of applications, including:

1. Genotoxicity testing: The assay is used to evaluate the genotoxic potential of various substances, including pharmaceuticals, environmental pollutants, and dietary components.

2. Cancer research: By assessing the frequency of micronuclei in lymphocytes, researchers can identify individuals at higher risk for cancer due to genetic predispositions or environmental exposures.

3. Radiation sensitivity: The assay can help predict individual responses to radiation therapy, allowing for personalized treatment plans based on a patient's cellular response to DNA damage.

4. Nutrigenomics: The CBMN assay is also applied in studies examining the effects of dietary components on DNA integrity and repair mechanisms.

2.2.3.3 Advantages of the CBMN assay

1. Sensitivity: The assay is highly sensitive and can detect low levels of DNA damage, making it suitable for biomonitoring studies.

2. Relevance: Since lymphocytes are easily accessible and reflect systemic exposure to genotoxic agents, the results are relevant to human health.

3. Comprehensive assessment: The assay provides a comprehensive assessment of cellular responses, including cytotoxicity, cell proliferation, and DNA damage.

2.2.3.4 Challenges and considerations

1. Technical variability: The assay requires careful attention to detail in each step to minimize variability. Factors such as cell density, culture conditions, and staining protocols can influence results.

2. Interpretation of results: The presence of micronuclei can be influenced by various factors, including cell cycle stage and individual genetic differences. Therefore, results should be interpreted in the context of other biological data.

3. Ethical considerations: The use of human lymphocytes necessitates ethical considerations regarding sample collection and informed consent.

The cytokinesis-block micronucleus cytome assay is a valuable method for assessing DNA damage and cellular responses to genotoxic agents. The detailed protocol provided in the article serves as a comprehensive guide for researchers looking to implement this assay in their studies. By understanding the methodology, applications, and implications of the CBMN assay, scientists can contribute to advancing knowledge in fields such as cancer research, environmental health, and personalized medicine.

As research continues to evolve, the CBMN assay remains a critical tool for understanding the complexities of DNA damage and repair, ultimately aiding in the development of strategies for cancer prevention and treatment.

Apart from these tests, number of other traditional cytotoxicity assays have been discovered and been in use such as the chromium release test, model cavity test, neutral red uptake assay, and Millipore filter test (**Table 1**).

2.3 Cytotoxicity and cell death

Cell death is an essential biological process that occurs in a multitude of contexts, ranging from the development of organisms to the maintenance of tissue homeostasis. Cells can cease to function in various ways, and understanding these mechanisms is crucial to grasping how organisms regulate life and death at the cellular level. Below, we explore the primary types of cell death and their implications.

2.3.1 Apoptosis (type I cell death)

Apoptosis can be likened to a graceful ballet of cellular demise, representing a highly regulated form of programmed cell death (PCD). This process occurs in a controlled manner and is independent of external stimuli, emphasizing the intrinsic mechanisms of cellular regulation. The initiation of apoptosis is dictated by biochemical signals encoded within the cell's DNA, which orchestrate a well-defined pathway leading to self-destruction [19].

Method	Advantages	Limitations	Application	References
Development of oncolytic viruses	Can be used in immunotherapy for cancer treatment	Selection of oncolytic viruses, virus entry and selection	Treatment of cancer	[10, 11]
Foam separation	Easy and simple downstream process	Can be used for specific proteins only, limits the use to certain concentrations of proteins	Separation of hydrophobic and thermostable enzymes	[12]
Ozone based method	Can be used for temperature-sensitive proteins	Can only be used for bacterial and algae	Integrated process for detection and lysis of cells	[13]
Monolith columns	Can be used for large size proteins	Not suitable for small size proteins	Lysis of yeasts	[14, 15]
Microwave	Rapid and ease of scale-up	Not much cost effective, may lead to formation of free radicals	Can be widely utilized for algal cells	[16]
Nanoparticles based methods	Less toxic to the proteins and lipids	Specificity is higher as compared to other methods, and development and availability of nanoparticles is another issue.	Can be widely used in lysis of mammalian cells	[17]
Bacterial mediated	Specific and targeted cell lysis	Time-consuming and requires continuous monitoring of bacterial growth	Can be used for the extraction of temperature-sensitive proteins	[18]

Table 1.
Recent developments in the innovative approaches for cell lysis.

2.3.1.1 Triggers of apoptosis

The onset of apoptosis can be triggered by a variety of factors, both internal and external to the cell. Internal triggers may include mild cellular injury or stress, while external cues could involve signals related to developmental processes or the withdrawal of survival signals. These factors signal the cell to commence the apoptotic process, ensuring that cellular turnover is maintained [20].

2.3.1.2 The process of apoptosis

During apoptosis, cells undergo a series of morphological changes. Initially, the cell will shrink and lose its characteristic shape, which is a hallmark of this process. The cell's internal structure begins to break down, leading to distinct features such as chromatin condensation and the fragmentation of the nucleus. Ultimately, these changes result in the formation of apoptotic bodies, which are then phagocytosed by neighboring cells or immune cells, ensuring that the remnants of the dying cell are efficiently removed without eliciting an inflammatory response.

DOI: http://dx.doi.org/10.5772/intechopen.1008313

2.3.1.3 Importance of apoptosis

Apoptosis plays a vital role in the development and maintenance of multicellular organisms. This process is crucial for controlled growth, proper development, and the ongoing turnover of cells within tissues. A classic example of apoptosis in action can be observed during embryonic development, where it facilitates the separation of digits in the developing hands and feet. By selectively eliminating cells, apoptosis contributes to the formation of functional structures and helps to sculpt the organism.

2.3.1.4 Mechanisms of apoptosis

To date, two primary pathways have been identified in the process of apoptosis: the extrinsic pathway and the intrinsic pathway. The extrinsic pathway is activated by the engagement of death receptors on the cell surface, while the intrinsic pathway is governed by mitochondrial enzymes that play a pivotal role in the apoptotic process. These pathways highlight the complexity and precision with which cells regulate their own demise [21].

2.3.2 Autophagy (type II cell death)

Autophagy can be viewed as a form of cellular spring cleaning, where cells actively degrade and recycle their own components. This process involves the engulfment of organelles and cytoplasmic contents, which are then directed to lysosomes for degradation. Depending on the context, autophagy can serve dual functions: promoting cell survival under nutrient-limited conditions or facilitating cell death when cellular damage is extensive.

2.3.2.1 The autophagic process

During autophagy, cells essentially take stock of their internal components, identifying worn-out organelles and misfolded proteins that require removal. This self-eating process not only cleans up cellular debris but also recycles essential components to support cellular metabolism and energy production. Thus, autophagy plays a critical role in maintaining cellular health and homeostasis [22].

2.3.3 Necrosis (type III cell death)

Necrosis has historically been regarded as the chaotic and uncontrolled cousin of cell death, often resulting from acute cellular injury. However, recent research has illuminated specific pathways of regulated necrosis that add complexity to this process. Unlike apoptosis, necrosis typically occurs in response to severe stress or injury, leading to cell swelling and eventual rupture [23].

2.3.3.1 Regulated necrosis pathways

Within the umbrella of necrosis, several distinct pathways have been identified:

- *Necroptosis:* This is a programmed form of necrosis that occurs when cells experience certain signals, often when apoptosis is inhibited. It involves receptor-interacting protein kinases (RIPKs) that promote cell death in a regulated manner.

- *Pyroptosis:* This is characterized by inflammatory cell death, primarily in response to infections. Pyroptosis leads to the release of pro-inflammatory cytokines, making it a crucial response in the immune system.

- *Ferroptosis:* This pathway involves iron-dependent lipid peroxidation, leading to cell death that is distinct from other forms of necrosis. Ferroptosis has garnered attention for its implications in various diseases, including cancer.

- *NETosis:* This is a unique form of cell death observed in neutrophils, where they release extracellular traps composed of DNA and antimicrobial proteins. This process helps to trap and eliminate pathogens but can also contribute to tissue damage if dysregulated.

3. Challenges in cell lysis

3.1 Challenges in physical and chemical methods of cell lysis

Most of the bioproducts are needed to be extracted before proceeding toward purification. Since the products are mostly intracellular, the cell wall and/or cell membrane need to be ruptured for release of products in crude form. One of the basic methods for the rupturing of cells is physical and chemical-based methods. Depending upon the nature and properties of the product and its source of production, cell lysis methods are decided. Many processes involve single-step procedures while others may involve a cascade of multiple procedures for efficient extraction. However, these methods often come with several limitations which one has to deal with while implying or integrating in the bioprocessing platforms.

The bead mill method is one of the oldest mechanical methods of cell disruption. It heavily depends on the cell type be it bacterial, yeast or plant, and the nature of the cell wall. It involves mild to heavy grinding of the cells. The grinding process is done by using microbeads, and its size and weight depend on the cell type and its vulnerability to disruption. One of the limitations is the heat generation process. As the bead size increases, the heat generation also increases which may affect the stability of the desired product. The limitation is backed up by poor recovery and poor scale-up [24].

Ultrasonication is another cell disruption method which is used for cell lysis. There are two ways to perform a cell lysis using sonication. One is the water bath method, and the other is the dip probe method. While water bath sonication is a very mild method of sonication, the dip probe method is a more efficient method for the recovery of biological products. These are mostly used for bacterial and yeast-based products. The method is used in combination with any other physical or chemical methods [1]. However, it also has serious limitations such as poor scale-up and high energy usage, another major limitation to this is that the process requires a separate area as the ultrasonic waves pose a health hazard [1].

Thermolysis and osmotic shock are the methods which do not involve mechanical setup; however, these are also physical-based methods. Thermolysis involves the treatment of cells at high temperatures causing cell disruption. For effective disruption, a cold cycle may be integrated, but this leads to limitations of poor recovery. One of the important things to note here is that temperature variation may change the properties of the desired biological product, especially in the case of enzymes which become highly critical. One of the lysis methods is osmotic shock which involves the treatment of cells with high and low-salt solutions in a disruptive manner. The disruption causes the development of osmotic pressure across the membranes disrupting the cell membranes. This method is utilized in biopharmaceutical and biotechnological processes, but the yield and inefficiency serve as limitations of this method [25].

Chemical methods of cell lysis involve the use of detergents and enzymes for cellular disruption. Chemicals such as Sodium dodecyl sulfate (SDS), TritonX-100, and Tween- 80, etc. are also used. The detergents interact with the receptors on the cell membrane and lead to membrane damage. They work by solubilizing the membrane proteins and thereby creating space for the release of cellular components. While the use of chemicals leads to issues with the recovery and stability of the desired compounds, the enzymatic methods such as lysozymes and peptidases cause issues with the recovery of the biological products as their activity may lead to the inactivity of the biomolecules [26].

Another approach utilized for cell lysis is the use of solvents for extraction and cell disruption, while this approach is widely utilized in the case of natural products from plants as the cell wall has a significant resistance to the solvents. Organic solvents such as ether, methanol, chloroform, etc. are used. This method is accompanied by the limitations of product stability and additional downstream costs due to solvent removal and recovery steps [26].

4. Development of innovative cell lysis approaches

To overcome the limitations of the traditional cell lysis methods, we need to focus on developing new roads to the development of lysis techniques.

1. Nanotechnology: The use of nanoparticles for cell lysis is a promising area of research. For instance, Seo et al. [27] developed octahedral $ZnFe_2O_4$ nanoparticles that act as magnetic flocculants, enabling simultaneous harvesting and lysis of microalgal cells. These nanoparticles can be functionalized to enhance their lytic capabilities, allowing for targeted disruption of specific cell types.

2. Microfluidic devices: Advances in microfluidics have led to the development of devices that can achieve cell lysis through mechanical means. Yun et al. [28] created a microfluidic device with ultra-sharp nano-blades that apply shear forces to disrupt cell membranes. This method allows for precise control over the lysis process and can be scaled for high-throughput applications, making it suitable for various research and clinical settings.

3. Molecular dynamics simulations: Capozza et al. [29] conducted in-silico studies to understand the behavior of cell membranes under mechanical stress. Their findings suggest that creating curvature in the membrane can significantly reduce the force required for lysis, paving the way for more efficient mechanical lysis techniques. This approach can inform the design of new lysis devices that optimize the mechanical forces applied to cells.

4. Laser-based methods: Pulsed laser microbeam techniques have been explored for cell lysis, where focused laser beams induce localized heating and pressure changes, leading to cell disruption. This method allows for precise targeting of specific cells without affecting surrounding tissues, making it a valuable tool for applications in single-cell analysis and tissue engineering [30].

5. Acoustic lysis: This method utilizes ultrasonic waves to create cavitation bubbles in the surrounding medium, which collapse and generate shock waves that disrupt cell membranes. Acoustic lysis is effective for lysing various cell types, including bacteria, yeast, and mammalian cells.

Despite the advancements in cell lysis technologies, several challenges remain. The review identifies issues such as the need for methods that are gentle enough to preserve sensitive biomolecules while still being effective at lysing cells. Additionally, scalability and cost-effectiveness are critical factors that need to be addressed for widespread adoption of new technologies (**Figure 1**) [31].

Future research directions include:

1. *Hybrid methods*: The development of hybrid methods that combine physical, chemical, and biological approaches to achieve optimal lysis efficiency. For example, combining enzymatic lysis with mechanical disruption could enhance the overall lysis process while minimizing damage to sensitive biomolecules.

2. *Artificial intelligence and machine learning*: There is a growing interest in exploring the use of artificial intelligence and machine learning to optimize lysis protocols based on specific cell types and applications. These technologies can analyze large datasets to identify the most effective lysis conditions, leading to more efficient and tailored lysis strategies.

3. *Nanostructured materials*: Continued research into nanostructured materials for cell lysis could lead to the development of new lysis agents that are more effective and selective. For instance, nanoparticles that can be targeted to specific

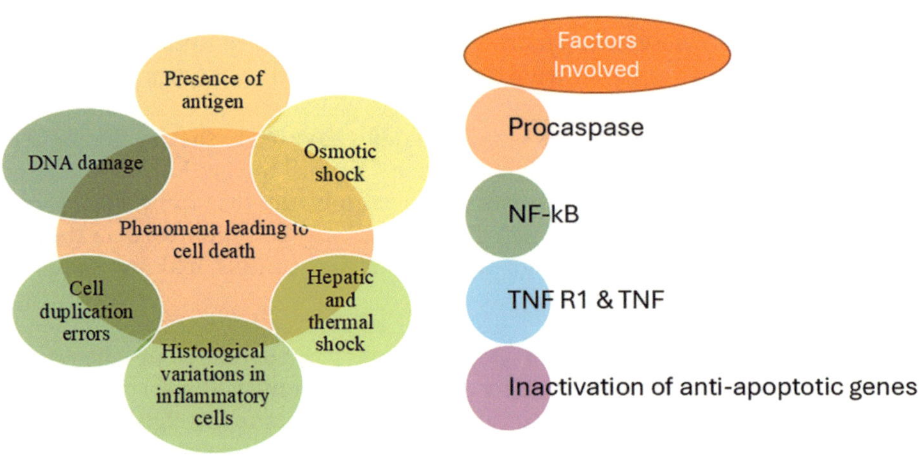

Figure 1.
Incidents that induce cell death and some of the cellular factors associated with it.

cell types or that respond to external stimuli (e.g., light or temperature) could enhance the precision of lysis methods.

4. *Integration with other techniques*: Integrating cell lysis methods with downstream applications, such as nucleic acid extraction and analysis, could streamline workflows and improve overall efficiency. For example, developing lysis methods that are compatible with microfluidic platforms could facilitate the automation of sample processing.

Acknowledgements

We acknowledge the use of ChatGPT for language polishing of the manuscript.

Author details

Pragya Prakash[1], Shoaib Haidar[1] and Hare Ram Singh[2*]

1 Centre for Biopharmaceutical Technology, Department of Chemical Engineering, Indian Institute of Technology, Delhi, India

2 Department of Biotechnology and Bio-Engineering, Birla Institute of Technology Mesra, Ranchi, India

*Address all correspondence to: hrsingh@bitmesra.ac.in

References

[1] Gomes TA, Zanette CM, Spier MR. An overview of cell disruption methods for intracellular biomolecules recovery. Preparative Biochemistry and Biotechnology. 2020;**50**(7):635-654

[2] Minute L, Teijeira A, Sanchez-Paulete AR, Ochoa MC, Alvarez M, Otano I, et al. Cellular cytotoxicity is a form of immunogenic cell death. Journal for Immunotherapy of Cancer. 2020;**8**(1):1-13

[3] Salih Istifli E, Basri Ila H, editors. Cytotoxicity - Definition, Identification, and Cytotoxic Compounds [Internet]. London, UK: IntechOpen; 2019

[4] Shehadul Islam M, Aryasomayajula A, Selvaganapathy PR. A review on macroscale and microscale cell lysis methods. Micromachines. 2017;**8**(3):83

[5] Çelik TA. Introductory chapter: Cytotoxicity. In: Cytotoxicity. London, UK: InTech; 2018

[6] Keech BH, McCaroll B, Farrow MG. Alternatives to polyvinyl chloride as the positive control material for tissue culture agar overlay assay. In: Transactions of the 9th Annual Meeting of the Society for Biomaterials. Vol. 69. Birmingham, Alabama; 1983

[7] Ghasemi M, Turnbull T, Sebastian S, Kempson I. The MTT assay: Utility, limitations, pitfalls, and interpretation in bulk and single-cell analysis. International Journal of Molecular Sciences. 2021;**22**(23):12827

[8] Carreño EA, Alberto AV, de Souza CA, de Mello HL, Henriques-Pons A, Anastacio AL. Considerations and technical pitfalls in the employment of the MTT assay to evaluate photosensitizers for photodynamic therapy. Applied Sciences. 2021;**11**(6):2603

[9] Fenech M. Cytokinesis-block micronucleus cytome assay. Nature Protocols. 2007;**2**(5):1084-1104

[10] Hensten-Pettersen A. Comparison of the methods available for assessing cytotoxicity. International Endodontic Journal. 1988;**21**(2):89-99

[11] Abd-Aziz N, Poh CL. Development of oncolytic viruses for cancer therapy. Translational Research. Nov 2021;**237**:98-123

[12] Fang S, Huang W, Wu J, Han J, Wang L, Wang Y. Separation and purification of recombinant β-glucosidase with hydrophobicity and thermally responsive property from cell lysis solution by foam separation and further purification. Journal of Agricultural and Food Chemistry. 2023;**71**(7):3362-3372

[13] Lee EH, Lim HJ, Son A, Chua B. A disposable bacterial lysis cartridge (BLC) suitable for an in situ water-borne pathogen detection system. The Analyst. 2015;**140**(22):7776-7783

[14] Aly MA, Nguon O, Gauthier M, Yeow JT. Antibacterial porous polymeric monolith columns with amphiphilic and polycationic character on cross-linked PMMA substrates for cell lysis applications. RSC Advances. 2013;**3**(46):24177-24184

[15] Aly Saad Aly M, Gauthier M, Yeow J. On-chip cell lysis by antibacterial non-leaching reusable quaternary ammonium monolithic column. Biomedical Microdevices. 2016;**18**:1-3

[16] Yun EJ, Kim HT, Cho KM, Yu S, Kim S, Choi IG, et al. Pretreatment and saccharification of red macroalgae to produce fermentable sugars. Bioresource Technology. Jan 2016;**199**:311-318

[17] Corredor C, Hou WC, Klein SA, Moghadam BY, Goryll M, Doudrick K, et al. Disruption of model cell membranes by carbon nanotubes. Carbon. 2013;**60**:67-75

[18] Wang M, Chen S, Zhou W, Yuan W, Wang D. Algal cell lysis by bacteria: A review and comparison to conventional methods. Algal Research. 2020;**46**:101794

[19] Obeng E. Apoptosis (programmed cell death) and its signals—A review. Brazilian Journal of Biology. 2020;**81**(4):1133-1143

[20] Li S, Ma Y, Ye S, Tang S, Liang N, Liang Y, et al. Polystyrene microplastics trigger hepatocyte apoptosis and abnormal glycolytic flux via ROS-driven calcium overload. Journal of Hazardous Materials. 2021;**417**:126025

[21] Ulukaya E, Acilan C, Yilmaz Y. Apoptosis: Why and how does it occur in biology? Cell Biochemistry and Function. 2011;**29**(6):468-480

[22] Denton D, Kumar S. Autophagy-dependent cell death. Cell Death and Differentiation. 2019;**26**(4):605-616

[23] Fink SL, Cookson BT. Apoptosis, pyroptosis, and necrosis: Mechanistic description of dead and dying eukaryotic cells. Infection and Immunity. 2005;**73**(4):1907-1916

[24] Tanaka H, Ochii Y, Moroto Y, Hirata D, Ibaraki T, Ogawara KI. Optimization of milling parameters for low metal contamination in bead milling technology. BPB Reports. 2022;**5**(3):45-49

[25] Koschorreck K, Wahrendorff F, Biemann S, Jesse A, Urlacher VB. Cell thermolysis—A simple and fast approach for isolation of bacterial laccases with potential to decolorize industrial dyes. Process Biochemistry. 2017;**56**:171-176

[26] Kakko N, Ivanona N, Rantasalo A. Cell disruption methods. In: CHEM-E3140 Bioprocess Technology II. 2016. pp. 11-13

[27] Seo JY, Jeon HJ, Kim JW, Lee J, Oh YK, Ahn CW, et al. Simulated-sunlight-driven cell lysis of magnetophoretically separated microalgae using ZnFe2O4 octahedrons. Industrial and Engineering Chemistry Research. 2018;**57**(5):1655-1661

[28] Yun SS, Yoon SY, Song MK, Im SH, Kim S, Lee JH, et al. Handheld mechanical cell lysis chip with ultra-sharp silicon nano-blade arrays for rapid intracellular protein extraction. Lab on a Chip. 2010;**10**(11):1442-1446

[29] Capozza R, Caprettini V, Gonano CA, Bosca A, Moia F, Santoro F, et al. Cell membrane disruption by vertical micro-/nanopillars: Role of membrane bending and traction forces. ACS Applied Materials and Interfaces. 2018;**10**(34):29107-29114

[30] Gazor M, Talesh SS, Kavianpour A, Khatami M, Javidanbardan A, Hosseini SN. A novel cell disruption approach: Effectiveness of laser-induced cell lysis of *Pichia pastoris* in the continuous system. Biotechnology and Bioprocess Engineering. 2018;**23**:49-54

[31] Mutafopulos K, Lu PJ, Garry R, Spink P, Weitz DA. Selective cell encapsulation, lysis, pico-injection and size-controlled droplet generation using traveling surface acoustic waves in a microfluidic device. Lab on a Chip. 2020;**20**(21):3914-3921

Chapter 7

Comparative Analysis of Cytotoxicity Assays, from Traditional to Modern Approaches

Mitali Singhal, Sabita Shaha and Maria Katsikogianni

Abstract

This chapter will provide a comprehensive comparative analysis of various cytotoxicity assays, including traditional methods like the MTT assay and modern approaches such as the ATP assay and flow cytometry. Each method will be examined in detail, covering its principle, procedure, advantages, limitations, and specific applications in cytotoxicity testing. Additionally, the chapter will address the interconnectivity of different cell death pathways—apoptosis, autophagy, and necrosis—and discuss how various assays can be used in combination to achieve a more accurate and holistic assessment of cell viability and death mechanisms. Practical guidelines will be provided to help researchers select the most appropriate assay based on their specific experimental requirements, cell types, and research objectives. By offering a comparative framework, this chapter aims to equip researchers with the knowledge needed to enhance the accuracy and reliability of their cytotoxicity assessments, ultimately advancing toxicological research and drug development.

Keywords: cytotoxicity assays, MTT assay, LDH assay, ATP assay, flow cytometry, cell viability

1. Introduction

1.1 Overview of cytotoxicity and its importance

Cytotoxicity refers to the quality of being toxic to cells. It is a crucial parameter in various fields of biological research, particularly in toxicology, pharmacology, and biomedical sciences [1, 2]. The primary goal of cytotoxicity testing is to evaluate the extent to which substances such as chemicals, pharmaceutical compounds, or environmental agents can harm or kill cells. For instance, cytotoxicity assays may produce variable results when applied to complex cell models like organoids, which are three-dimensional structures that mimic real tissue environments [3]. Cytotoxicity assays are used in basic research and drug discovery to identify toxic compounds on potential cancer therapeutics [4].

1.2 Understanding cytotoxicity is essential for several reasons

1.2.1 Drug development and safety assessment

In the pharmaceutical industry, cytotoxicity assays are integral to the drug development process. Assessing the cytotoxicity of potential drug candidates is a critical step in ensuring their safety and efficacy. They help identify potential toxic effects of new drug candidates early in the development pipeline, ensuring that only safe and effective compounds progress to clinical trials. This not only protects patients but also reduces the risk of costly late-stage failures.

1.2.2 Toxicological research

Cytotoxicity testing is a cornerstone of toxicological studies, which aim to understand the adverse effects of various substances on living organisms. By assessing the cytotoxic potential of chemicals, researchers can predict their impact on human health and the environment. This is particularly important for regulatory purposes, where safety standards must be met to prevent harm to humans and ecosystems.

1.2.3 Biomedical research and therapeutics

In the realm of biomedical research, cytotoxicity assays are used to investigate the mechanisms of cell death and survival. This is vital for understanding diseases characterized by uncontrolled cell growth, such as cancer, or excessive cell death, as seen in neurodegenerative disorders. Moreover, cytotoxicity assessments are critical for developing and testing new therapeutic strategies, including chemotherapy, radiation therapy, and targeted therapies.

1.2.4 Product safety and quality control

Beyond pharmaceuticals, cytotoxicity testing is also relevant for the safety and quality control of various consumer products, including cosmetics, food additives, and household chemicals. Ensuring that these products are non-toxic to human cells is essential for protecting public health.

1.2.5 Environmental and occupational health

Cytotoxicity testing plays a key role in environmental and occupational health studies. By evaluating the toxic effects of environmental pollutants and workplace chemicals on cells, researchers can identify and mitigate potential health risks, leading to the implementation of safer practices and regulations.

In summary, cytotoxicity testing is a fundamental aspect of scientific research that bridges multiple disciplines. Its importance lies in safeguarding human health, advancing medical knowledge, ensuring the safety and efficacy of new drugs, and protecting the environment. This chapter aims to provide a comprehensive analysis of various cytotoxicity assays, comparing traditional and modern approaches to offer researchers a robust framework for accurate and reliable cytotoxicity assessment.

2. Objective and scope of the chapter

The primary objective of this chapter is to provide a comprehensive comparative analysis of various cytotoxicity assays, highlighting both traditional methods and modern approaches. By examining the principles, procedures, advantages, limitations, and specific applications of these assays, this chapter aims to equip researchers with the knowledge needed to select the most appropriate methods for their experimental needs.

The scope of this chapter includes:

2.1 Detailed examination of cytotoxicity assays

A thorough review of traditional cytotoxicity assays includes the MTT assay, LDH release assay, and Trypan Blue exclusion assay. There is an exploration of modern cytotoxicity assays such as the ATP assay, flow cytometry, and caspase activity assays.

2.2 Comparative analysis

A comparative analysis of the different assays is carried out in terms of methodological differences, sensitivity, specificity, throughput, scalability, cost, resource requirements, data interpretation, and reproducibility.

2.3 Interconnectivity of cell death pathways

An in-depth discussion on the interconnected nature of cell death pathways includes apoptosis, autophagy, and necrosis. There is examination of how different assays can be used to assess these pathways and their interactions.

2.4 Combination of assays for enhanced accuracy

Strategies are for combining multiple assays to achieve a more comprehensive and accurate assessment of cell viability and death mechanisms. Case studies illustrate the benefits of using combined assay approaches.

2.5 Practical guidelines for researchers

Practical guidelines are to assist researchers in selecting the most appropriate cytotoxicity assays based on their specific experimental requirements, cell types, and research objectives. Best practices are carried out for assay implementation and troubleshooting common issues.

2.6 Future directions in cytotoxicity testing

There is an exploration of emerging technologies and innovations in cytotoxicity testing.

Discussion on the integration of cytotoxicity assays and their potential applications in personalized medicine. Identification of challenges and opportunities in the field of cytotoxicity testing.

3. Traditional cytotoxicity assays

(Principle, procedure, advantages, limitations, and applications in cytotoxicity testing).

3.1 MTT assay

The MTT assay is a colorimetric technique that measures cell metabolic activity, serving as an indicator of cell viability, proliferation, and cytotoxicity [5–7]. The assay is based on the reduction of the yellow tetrazolium salt (MTT) to purple formazan crystals by mitochondrial enzymes in viable cells, which occurs only in metabolically active cells. This makes the MTT assay a reliable method for assessing cell viability. MTT assays play a major role to examine the cytotoxicity of a drug [8, 9].

The procedure involves several steps. First, cells are seeded in a 96-well plate and allowed to adhere overnight. They are then treated with the test substance for a specified period. Following this, MTT solution is added to each well and incubated, typically for 1–4 hours, allowing viable cells to reduce MTT to formazan. After incubation, a solubilization solution, such as DMSO, is added to dissolve the formazan crystals. The absorbance of the resulting solution is then measured using a spectrophotometer at a wavelength of 570 nm, with a reference wavelength of 630 nm, correlating the absorbance with the number of viable cells.

The MTT assay has several advantages. It is simple and easy to perform, cost-effective due to inexpensive materials and reagents, and provides quantitative data on cell viability. Its wide applicability makes it suitable for various cell types and conditions. However, there are some limitations. As an end-point assay, it provides only a single time-point measurement, limiting its use for dynamic monitoring of cell viability. Compounds that affect mitochondrial function can interfere with the results, and inefficient dissolution of formazan crystals can lead to variability in readings. Additionally, the MTT reagent can be toxic to cells, potentially affecting cell viability during long incubation periods.

Despite these limitations, the MTT assay is widely used in various applications. It is frequently employed in drug screening to evaluate the cytotoxic effects of new drug candidates on cancer and normal cell lines. Toxicological studies assess the toxicity of chemicals, environmental agents, and nanoparticles. In biomedical research, it is used to investigate cell proliferation, apoptosis, and the effects of various treatments on cell viability. The assay is also compatible with 96- and 384-well formats, making it suitable for high-throughput screening applications.

In summary, the MTT assay is a robust, reliable, and widely used method for assessing cell viability and cytotoxicity, despite its limitations and potential interferences.

3.2 LDH release assay

The LDH release assay is a widely used method for assessing cell viability and cytotoxicity by measuring the release of lactate dehydrogenase (LDH) from damaged or lysed cells [10]. LDH is a stable cytoplasmic enzyme present in all cell types, and its release into the culture medium is a marker of cell membrane integrity and cell death. The principle of the assay is based on the conversion of lactate to pyruvate by LDH, coupled with the reduction of a tetrazolium salt to a colored formazan product, which can be quantified by measuring absorbance. It is used to assess the performance of the therapeutic efficacy of the *ex vivo* tumor models [11, 12].

The procedure involves first seeding cells in a culture plate and treating them with the test substance. After incubation, the supernatant containing released LDH is collected from each well. A reaction mixture containing lactate, NAD+, and a tetrazolium salt is added to the supernatant. The enzymatic reaction occurs, leading to the production of a colored formazan product, which is then measured using a spectrophotometer at a wavelength of 490 nm. The intensity of the color is proportional to the amount of LDH released, indicating the extent of cell damage.

The LDH release assay offers several advantages. It is a simple and rapid method that does not require cell lysis for measurement, allowing for the assessment of cell viability in real time. The assay is highly sensitive and can detect low levels of cell damage. It is also versatile, suitable for a wide range of cell types and experimental conditions. However, there are some limitations to consider. The assay measures total LDH activity in the medium, which can be affected by factors such as serum components and spontaneous LDH release from cells, potentially leading to background noise. Additionally, the assay is less specific for apoptosis compared to other methods that measure specific markers of cell death pathways.

Despite these limitations, the LDH release assay is extensively used in various applications. It is commonly employed in drug discovery and toxicology studies to evaluate the cytotoxic effects of compounds on different cell lines. In biomedical research, the assay is used to study mechanisms of cell injury and to assess the protective effects of potential therapeutic agents. The assay's ability to provide quantitative and real-time data makes it a valuable tool for high-throughput screening of cytotoxicity in a variety of experimental settings.

In summary, the LDH release assay is a reliable and efficient method for assessing cell viability and cytotoxicity. Its simplicity, sensitivity, and versatility make it a popular choice for researchers in toxicology, pharmacology, and biomedical sciences.

3.3 Trypan Blue exclusion assay

The Trypan Blue exclusion assay is a straightforward and widely used method for assessing cell viability and cytotoxicity by differentiating between live and dead cells. The principle of this assay relies on the ability of viable cells to exclude the Trypan Blue dye, whereas dead or damaged cells with compromised membrane integrity take up the dye and appear blue under a microscope. This differential staining allows for a clear distinction between live (unstained) and dead (blue-stained) cells [13].

The procedure involves first seeding the cells and treating them with the test substance. After incubation, a small volume of cell suspension is mixed with an equal volume of Trypan Blue solution and incubated for a few minutes. The mixture is then loaded onto a hemocytometer, and the cells are observed under a light microscope. Viable cells exclude the dye and remain clear, while non-viable cells absorb the dye and appear blue. The number of stained and unstained cells is counted, and the percentage of viable cells is calculated [13].

The Trypan Blue exclusion assay offers several advantages. It is simple, quick, and inexpensive, requiring minimal specialized equipment. The procedure can be easily performed and interpreted, making it accessible to researchers at all levels. Additionally, it provides immediate results and can be used with a variety of cell types. However, the assay also has limitations. It is subjective and can be prone to operator error, as it relies on manual counting under a microscope. The assay provides only a snapshot of cell viability at a single time point, and prolonged exposure to Trypan Blue can be toxic to cells, potentially affecting their viability.

Despite these limitations, the Trypan Blue exclusion assay is widely used in various applications. It is commonly employed in cell culture studies to assess cell viability after exposure to different treatments, such as drugs, toxins, or environmental stressors. The assay is also useful for routine monitoring of cell health and density in culture, ensuring optimal conditions for experiments. Furthermore, it serves as a rapid and cost-effective screening tool in preliminary cytotoxicity assessments before employing more sophisticated and quantitative methods.

In summary, the Trypan Blue exclusion assay is a practical and valuable method for evaluating cell viability and cytotoxicity. Its simplicity and ease of use make it a popular choice for researchers in cell biology, toxicology, and pharmacology, despite its inherent limitations.

4. Modern cytotoxicity assays

4.1 ATP assay

The ATP assay is a modern and highly sensitive method for assessing cell viability and cytotoxicity by measuring the amount of adenosine triphosphate (ATP) present in metabolically active cells. The principle of this assay is based on the fact that ATP is a key indicator of cellular energy status and viability. When cells are alive and metabolically active, they maintain high levels of ATP, whereas dead or dying cells show a significant reduction in ATP levels. The drop of ATP level in human blood cell is an indicative of high glucose [14]. The assay utilizes a luminescent reaction in which the enzyme luciferase catalyzes the conversion of luciferin to oxyluciferin in the presence of ATP, producing light. The intensity of the emitted light is directly proportional to the amount of ATP, and therefore, to the number of viable cells [15].

The procedure for the ATP assay involves several steps. First, cells are seeded in a multi-well plate and treated with the test substance. After the treatment period, an ATP-releasing reagent is added to lyse the cells and release their ATP content. Next, a luciferase-luciferin reagent is added, initiating the luminescent reaction. The plate is then read using a luminometer, which measures the light output. The luminescence data are analyzed to determine the viability of the cells, with higher luminescence indicating higher ATP levels and greater cell viability.

The ATP assay has several advantages. It is extremely sensitive and can detect very low levels of ATP, allowing for the detection of small changes in cell viability. The assay is also rapid and easy to perform, providing results within a short time frame. Additionally, it is suitable for high-throughput screening due to its compatibility with multi-well plate formats and automated luminometers. However, there are some limitations. The ATP assay can be affected by the presence of substances that interfere with the luciferase reaction or ATP stability. Additionally, the assay only measures ATP levels, which, while indicative of cell viability, do not provide information on the mechanisms of cell death.

Despite these limitations, the ATP assay is widely used in various applications. It is commonly employed in drug discovery and screening to evaluate the cytotoxic effects of new compounds on different cell lines. In toxicological studies, it is used to assess the impact of environmental toxins, chemicals, and other agents on cell viability. The assay is also valuable in biomedical research for investigating cellular responses to different treatments and conditions. Furthermore, its high sensitivity and rapid results make it an excellent choice for high-throughput screening in large-scale studies [2].

In summary, the ATP assay is a modern, sensitive, and efficient method for assessing cell viability and cytotoxicity. Its ease of use, rapid turnaround time, and compatibility with high-throughput screening make it a popular choice for researchers in various fields, including toxicology, pharmacology, and biomedical sciences.

4.2 Flow cytometry

Flow cytometry is a sophisticated and versatile method used for assessing cell viability and cytotoxicity by analyzing the physical and chemical characteristics of cells. The principle of flow cytometry involves the suspension of cells in a fluid stream, which is then passed through a laser beam. As cells pass through the laser, they scatter light and emit fluorescence (if stained with fluorescent dyes). Detectors capture these signals, allowing for the measurement of various parameters such as cell size, granularity, and fluorescence intensity, which can indicate cell viability, apoptosis, and other cellular events [16].

The procedure begins with the preparation of a single-cell suspension from the sample, followed by staining the cells with fluorescent dyes or antibodies that target specific cellular components. These dyes can indicate viability, apoptosis, or necrosis by binding to specific markers or penetrating cells with compromised membranes. The stained cells are then introduced into the flow cytometer, where they pass through a laser beam in single file. The emitted fluorescence and scattered light are detected and analyzed by the flow cytometer's software, generating data on the individual cells' characteristics. Flow cytometry is widely recognized for its ability to distinguish cells in solutions and is most commonly used for assessing peripheral blood, bone marrow, and other body fluids making it a staple in clinical and research settings [17].

4.3 Mass cytometers

Time-of-flight mass spectrometry and flow cytometry are combined to create a mass cytometer. Time-of-flight mass spectrometry employs heavy metal ion-tagged antibodies as a substitute for fluorescently tagged antibodies for cell identification. Usually, these antibodies belong to the lanthanide class [18]. There are methods such as methods, such as cell barcoding, could be employed to do this [19]. Furthermore, correction is unnecessary because the chemicals used in mass cytometry do not have the emission spectral overlap connected to fluorescent labels and cellular autofluoresce signals. The sample is destroyed during analysis, making cell sorting impossible, and the acquisition rate is much slower than that of a typical flow cytometer (1000 cells/second against 10,000 cells/second). Commercially available reagents currently cover 40 channels; however, this number will increase if more metal ions, such as platinum, are added for antibody conjugation [20].

4.4 Imaging flow cytometers (IFCs)

IFCs stand out by combining traditional flow cytometry with fluorescence microscopy. This unique blend allows for the rapid analysis of multi-parameter fluorescence and morphology at both the single-cell and population levels in a sample [18]. IFCs, like flow cytometers, can handle large cell numbers. However, they also have the ability to monitor the distribution of proteins within individual cells, a feature akin to a confocal or fluorescence microscope. This unique combination of features makes IFCs ideal for applications such as cell signaling, co-localization studies, cell-cell interactions, DNA damage and repair, and any other circumstance requiring the coordination of cellular location and fluorescence expression on a large number of cells [18].

Flow cytometry offers several advantages. It is highly sensitive and can analyze thousands of cells per second, providing statistically significant data from a single sample. The method is also capable of multi-parametric analysis, allowing researchers to assess multiple cellular characteristics simultaneously. Additionally, flow cytometry can distinguish between different cell populations within a heterogeneous sample, providing detailed insights into cell viability and death mechanisms. However, there are some limitations. The equipment is expensive and requires specialized training to operate. Sample preparation can be complex, and the assay requires a significant number of cells, which may not be available in all experiments.

Despite these limitations, flow cytometry is widely used in various applications. In drug discovery and toxicology, it is employed to evaluate the cytotoxic effects of compounds on different cell lines. The method is also valuable in immunology for characterizing immune cell subsets and their responses to treatments. In cancer research, flow cytometry is used to assess the efficacy of anticancer agents and to study tumor cell biology. Furthermore, it is used in clinical diagnostics to monitor disease progression and response to therapy in patients with conditions such as HIV and leukemia [21].

In summary, flow cytometry is a powerful and comprehensive method for assessing cell viability and cytotoxicity. Its ability to provide detailed, multi-parametric data on individual cells makes it an indispensable tool for researchers in various fields, including toxicology, pharmacology, immunology, and clinical diagnostics.

4.5 Caspase activity assay

The caspase activity assay is a precise and sensitive method used to assess cell viability and cytotoxicity by measuring the activity of caspases, which are crucial enzymes involved in the process of apoptosis. The principle of this assay is based on the detection of caspase activity through specific substrates that release a fluorescent or colorimetric signal upon cleavage by active caspases. This signal directly correlates with the level of apoptosis occurring within the cell population [22]. Notably, the assay can involve time-resolved fluorescence based on energy transfer from europium cryptate as a donor to cross-linked allophycocyanin as an acceptor (XL665), as demonstrated in earlier studies [23, 24].

The procedure typically involves treating cells with the test substance to induce apoptosis. After treatment, cells are lysed to release intracellular components, including caspases. A caspase-specific substrate, which is tagged with a fluorescent or chromogenic group, is then added to the cell lysate. Active caspases cleave the substrate, releasing the fluorescent or colored signal. This signal is measured using a fluorometer or spectrophotometer, providing a quantitative readout of caspase activity and, consequently, the extent of apoptosis.

The caspase activity assay offers several advantages. It is highly specific and sensitive, allowing for the detection of low levels of apoptosis. The assay provides quantitative results, making it easy to compare the effects of different treatments. Additionally, it can distinguish between various caspases by using substrates specific

DOI: http://dx.doi.org/10.5772/intechopen.1006842

to individual caspase types, offering insights into the specific apoptotic pathways activated. However, the assay has limitations. It requires cell lysis, which means it cannot provide real-time monitoring of apoptosis in live cells. Also, the presence of inhibitors or interfering substances in the sample can affect the accuracy of the results.

Despite these limitations, the caspase activity assay is widely used in various applications. It is commonly employed in drug discovery and toxicology to evaluate the pro-apoptotic or anti-apoptotic effects of compounds on different cell lines. In cancer research, it is used to study the mechanisms of action of anticancer agents and to identify potential therapeutic targets. The assay is also valuable in neuroscience for investigating neuronal apoptosis in response to neurotoxic stimuli. Furthermore, it is used in immunology to study apoptosis in immune cells and understand the regulation of immune responses.

In summary, the caspase activity assay is a powerful and specific method for assessing cell viability and cytotoxicity by measuring apoptosis. Its sensitivity, specificity, and quantitative nature make it an essential tool for researchers in various fields, including toxicology, pharmacology, cancer research, and immunology.

5. Comparative analysis of cytotoxicity assays

Comparative analysis of cytotoxicity assays involves examining the various methodologies, sensitivity, specificity, throughput, scalability, cost, resource requirements, data interpretation, and reproducibility of different assays. Each cytotoxicity assay employs unique methodologies to measure cell viability and death. For instance, the MTT assay relies on the reduction of tetrazolium salts to formazan by metabolically active cells, while the ATP assay measures the presence of ATP as an indicator of viable cells. Flow cytometry analyses multiple cellular characteristics simultaneously by detecting light scattering and fluorescence from stained cells, and the caspase activity assay specifically measures apoptosis by detecting caspase enzyme activity. These diverse methodologies cater to different experimental needs and provide varied insights into cell viability and death mechanisms.

In terms of sensitivity and specificity, modern assays such as the ATP and caspase activity assays tend to be more sensitive and specific compared to traditional methods like the Trypan Blue exclusion assay. The ATP assay can detect minute changes in ATP levels, providing highly sensitive measurements of cell viability. The caspase activity assay offers high specificity by targeting specific caspase enzymes involved in apoptosis. Traditional assays, while reliable, may lack the sensitivity and specificity needed for certain applications, making modern assays more suitable for detecting subtle cytotoxic effects.

Throughput and scalability are crucial factors in selecting an assay, particularly for high-throughput screening. Modern assays such as the ATP assay and flow cytometry are well-suited for high-throughput applications due to their ability to process numerous samples quickly and efficiently. Flow cytometry, for example, can analyze thousands of cells per second, making it highly scalable. In contrast, traditional assays such as the Trypan Blue exclusion assay and MTT assay, while straightforward and cost-effective, may not be as scalable for large-scale studies due to the need for manual counting or longer incubation times.

Cost and resource requirements vary among the assays. Traditional assays such as Trypan Blue and MTT are generally more cost-effective, requiring less expensive reagents and equipment. Modern assays, while offering higher sensitivity and throughput, often require more sophisticated equipment and reagents, increasing the overall cost. Flow cytometry, for instance, involves high initial investment in flow cytometers and requires specialized training to operate. The ATP and caspase activity assays, though more expensive than traditional methods, provide valuable data that justify the higher cost in many research settings.

Data interpretation and reproducibility are essential for reliable cytotoxicity testing. The simplicity of traditional assays such as the Trypan Blue exclusion assay allows for straightforward data interpretation, though they may be prone to operator variability. Modern assays like the ATP assay provide quantitative and easily interpretable results with higher reproducibility. Flow cytometry offers detailed, multi-parametric data, though it requires expertise in data analysis. The caspase activity assay provides specific insights into apoptosis, with reproducible results if performed correctly.

In summary, a comparative analysis of cytotoxicity assays highlights the strengths and limitations of each method. Modern assays, while more costly and complex, offer higher sensitivity, specificity, throughput, and scalability. Traditional assays, on the other hand, remain valuable for their simplicity, cost-effectiveness, and ease of interpretation. Researchers must consider these factors when choosing the most appropriate assay for their specific experimental needs.

6. Interconnectivity of cell death pathways

6.1 Apoptosis

Apoptosis is a programmed cell death mechanism that plays a crucial role in maintaining tissue homeostasis and eliminating damaged or unwanted cells. The disappearance of crucial cells within healthy tissues gives rise to the growth, progression, and treatment outcomes of many human disorders, including neurological and infectious diseases as well as environmental and medical toxicities [25]. The process is characterized by specific morphological and biochemical changes, including cell shrinkage, chromatin condensation, DNA fragmentation, and membrane blebbing. Apoptosis is regulated by two main pathways: the intrinsic (mitochondrial) pathway and the extrinsic (death receptor) pathway. The intrinsic pathway is triggered by internal signals such as DNA damage and involves the release of cytochrome c from mitochondria, leading to the activation of caspase-9. The extrinsic pathway is initiated by external signals binding to death receptors on the cell surface, resulting in the activation of caspase-8. Both pathways converge on the activation of executioner caspases, such as caspase-3, which carry out the dismantling of cellular components.

Key markers of apoptosis include the externalization of phosphatidylserine (detected by Annexin V staining), activation of caspases (measured by caspase activity assays), and the presence of DNA fragmentation (assessed by TUNEL assay or DNA laddering). Various assay methods are used to detect and quantify apoptosis, each targeting different aspects of the apoptotic process. Flow cytometry, for instance, can detect Annexin V binding and caspase activity, allowing for the analysis of large cell populations. The caspase activity assay specifically measures the enzymatic activity of caspases involved in apoptosis, providing quantitative data on the extent of cell death. Fluorescent and colorimetric assays, such as the TUNEL assay, identify DNA fragmentation, another hallmark of apoptosis.

In summary, apoptosis is a vital and tightly regulated process of programmed cell death with distinct mechanisms and markers. Assay methods targeting these markers are essential for studying apoptosis and understanding its role in various physiological and pathological conditions.

6.2 Autophagy

Autophagy is a catabolic process that plays a vital role in cellular homeostasis by degrading and recycling damaged organelles, misfolded proteins, and other intracellular components. Autophagy has a wide range of physiological and pathophysiological roles that are sometimes complex [26]. The mechanism of autophagy involves the formation of a double-membrane vesicle called the autophagosome, which engulfs the targeted cellular material. The autophagosome then fuses with a lysosome to form an autolysosome, where the contents are degraded by lysosomal enzymes. This process is regulated by a series of autophagy-related genes (ATGs) and key signaling pathways, such as the mTOR pathway, which inhibits autophagy in nutrient-rich conditions. Autophagy functionally transforms into various autophagy-mediated cell-killing mechanisms. For example, it can improve autophagy in disease therapy and offer a new perspective on tumor therapeutic treatment [27].

Key markers of autophagy include the conversion of the cytosolic protein LC3-I to the membrane-bound form LC3-II, which is associated with autophagosome formation. Another important marker is p62/SQSTM1, a protein that is selectively degraded during autophagy. The accumulation or reduction of these markers can be detected using Western blotting or immunofluorescence techniques. Additionally, the formation of autophagic vesicles can be visualized using electron microscopy, which provides detailed structural insights into the autophagic process [28, 29].

Various assay methods are employed to study autophagy. Fluorescence microscopy using GFP-LC3 or mCherry-LC3 fusion proteins allows for the visualization of autophagosome formation and dynamics in live cells. Flow cytometry can be used to quantify the level of autophagy by measuring the fluorescence intensity of autophagy markers. The use of specific inhibitors and activators of autophagy, combined with these detection methods, enables researchers to dissect the regulatory mechanisms and functional roles of autophagy in different cellular contexts.

In summary, autophagy is a crucial cellular process for maintaining homeostasis through the degradation and recycling of intracellular components. Key markers like LC3-II and p62, along with various assay methods, provide valuable tools for studying the mechanisms and regulation of autophagy, enhancing our understanding of its role in health and disease.

6.3 Necrosis

Necrosis is a form of cell death characterized by uncontrolled and detrimental cellular damage, often resulting from acute injury or severe stress [30, 31]. Unlike apoptosis, which is a programmed and regulated process, necrosis is typically associated with cellular swelling, loss of membrane integrity, and the subsequent release of intracellular contents into the extracellular space [32]. This uncontrolled release can trigger inflammatory responses and damage surrounding tissues. The mechanisms underlying necrosis often involve disruptions in cellular ion homeostasis, mitochondrial dysfunction, and oxidative stress [33].

Key markers of necrosis include the loss of plasma membrane integrity, which can be detected using vital dyes like Trypan blue or propidium iodide, which penetrate damaged cells and stain their contents. Additionally, the release of intracellular enzymes, such as lactate dehydrogenase (LDH), into the extracellular medium is a common indicator of necrosis. LDH release assays are widely used to quantify cell membrane damage and assess the extent of necrotic cell death [34].

Assay methods for studying necrosis typically focus on detecting cell membrane integrity and measuring the release of intracellular components. The LDH release assay measures the activity of LDH in the culture supernatant, providing a quantitative assessment of necrotic cell death. Trypan Blue exclusion and propidium iodide staining are employed to visualize and quantify necrotic cells under a microscope. Additionally, assays that measure the release of other intracellular molecules, such as high mobility group box 1 protein (HMGB1), can provide further insights into necrotic processes.

In summary, necrosis is an uncontrolled form of cell death associated with significant cellular and tissue damage. Key markers such as loss of membrane integrity and LDH release, along with various assay methods, are essential for understanding the mechanisms and consequences of necrosis, thereby advancing research into its role in disease and potential therapeutic interventions.

6.4 Cross-talk between pathways

The cross-talk between cell death pathways—apoptosis, autophagy, and necrosis—reveals a complex network of interactions that significantly influence cellular responses to stress and damage. These pathways do not operate in isolation; rather, they can exhibit synergistic or antagonistic interactions that impact the overall outcome of cytotoxicity testing. For instance, during cellular stress, apoptosis and autophagy can be interconnected, with autophagic activity sometimes preceding or facilitating apoptosis. Conversely, excessive autophagy can lead to a type of cell death that shares characteristics with necrosis, especially when cellular damage is severe and exceeds the cell's ability to repair.

In terms of synergy, autophagy can act as a protective mechanism by removing damaged organelles and proteins, thereby delaying apoptosis and preventing necrosis. However, if the stress continues or escalates, this initially protective role can shift to become a contributor to cell death. On the other hand, certain conditions might promote necrosis when apoptosis is impaired or overwhelmed, leading to a more inflammatory response.

Antagonistic interactions are also evident; for example, anti-apoptotic signals can inhibit apoptotic pathways while simultaneously affecting autophagy. This cross-talk complicates the interpretation of cytotoxicity tests, as the presence of multiple cell death pathways and their interactions can influence the outcomes of assays and the effectiveness of therapeutic interventions. Understanding these interactions is crucial for accurate cytotoxicity testing, as it helps in predicting how cells might respond to various treatments and in designing more effective strategies for targeting specific cell death pathways in disease contexts.

Overall, the interplay between different cell death pathways underscores the importance of a comprehensive approach in cytotoxicity testing, considering how these pathways influence each other and contribute to the overall cell fate.

7. Combining assays for enhanced assessment

Combining multiple cytotoxicity assays can provide a more comprehensive and nuanced understanding of cell viability and death mechanisms, overcoming the limitations inherent in any single method. The rationale for using a combination of assays lies in the diverse nature of cell death processes and the varying insights each assay offers. For example, while the MTT assay measures metabolic activity, it does not distinguish between apoptosis and necrosis. In contrast, the caspase activity assay specifically targets apoptotic pathways, and the LDH release assay provides insights into membrane integrity and necrosis. By integrating these assays, researchers can capture a fuller picture of the cytotoxic effects of a compound, including its impact on different cell death pathways.

Several case studies illustrate the effectiveness of combined assay approaches. For instance, combining the ATP assay with flow cytometry can simultaneously provide quantitative data on cell viability and detailed insights into cell populations and death mechanisms. Another example includes using the Trypan Blue exclusion assay in conjunction with the LDH release assay to cross-validate results and gain a clearer understanding of both membrane integrity and overall cell viability. These combined approaches enhance the accuracy of cytotoxicity assessments and can reveal subtle effects that might be missed with a single assay.

When selecting assays, researchers should consider several factors to tailor their choice to specific experimental needs. Optimal assay selection involves evaluating the specific research objectives, the type of cell death being studied, and the experimental context. For example, if the focus is on understanding apoptotic pathways, combining caspase activity assays with Annexin V staining may be appropriate. If the goal is to assess broad cytotoxic effects and differentiate between multiple forms of cell death, using a combination of MTT, LDH, and flow cytometry might be more suitable.

Practical guidelines for assay selection should consider factors such as assay sensitivity, specificity, cost, and resource requirements. Researchers should also take into account the scale of their study, whether high-throughput screening is needed, and the type of cells being used. Customizing assay choices based on these parameters ensures that the selected assays align with the experimental goals and provide the most relevant and reliable data for interpreting cytotoxicity.

In summary, combining multiple assays offers a more comprehensive assessment of cytotoxicity by integrating various perspectives on cell viability and death mechanisms. Effective assay selection involves careful consideration of research needs, assay characteristics, and practical constraints, enabling researchers to achieve accurate and meaningful results in their cytotoxicity studies.

8. Best practices for assay implementation

Implementing cytotoxicity assays effectively requires adherence to best practices to ensure reliable and reproducible results. First and foremost, proper experimental design is crucial, including the use of appropriate controls, replication, and randomization to account for variability and minimize bias. Researchers should carefully select and calibrate equipment to maintain accuracy and consistency in measurements. Additionally, the choice of assays should be tailored to the specific research objectives, considering the type of cell death being investigated and the sensitivity required for detection.

Standardizing sample preparation and handling procedures is another key aspect of best practices. Cells should be cultured under consistent conditions, and treatments should be applied uniformly to avoid variability. For assays involving staining or labeling, it is important to follow established protocols and optimize reagent concentrations to achieve reliable and interpretable results.

Data analysis also plays a critical role in assay implementation. Employing appropriate statistical methods to analyze the data helps ensure that the results are statistically valid and meaningful. Researchers should also be mindful of potential sources of error, such as interference from assay reagents or contaminants, and take steps to mitigate these issues.

Finally, documenting and reporting experimental procedures and results transparently is essential for reproducibility and comparison across studies. Providing detailed methodology and acknowledging any limitations allows for more accurate interpretation and facilitates the validation of findings by other researchers.

In summary, best practices for conducting cytotoxicity assays include rigorous experimental design, standardized procedures, accurate data analysis, and transparent reporting. Adhering to these practices enhances the reliability and reproducibility of results, ultimately advancing the quality and impact of cytotoxicity research.

8.1 Troubleshooting common issues

Troubleshooting common issues in cytotoxicity testing is essential for obtaining accurate and reliable results. One frequent problem is inconsistent or unexpected assay results, which can often be traced back to issues with sample preparation or assay execution. Ensuring that cells are cultured under optimal conditions and that treatments are applied uniformly can help mitigate variability. Additionally, checking the expiration dates and proper storage of reagents can prevent issues related to reagent degradation, which may affect assay performance.

Another common issue is interference from assay reagents or contamination. To address this, researchers should include appropriate controls and verify that reagents do not interact with the assay components in unintended ways. For assays requiring cell staining or labeling, ensuring that the staining protocols are followed accurately and that cells are properly fixed or permeabilized is crucial for obtaining reliable data.

Inconsistent results can also arise from equipment malfunctions or calibration errors. Regular maintenance and calibration of equipment, such as spectrophotometers or flow cytometers, are essential to maintain accuracy. If equipment issues are suspected, recalibrating or replacing faulty components may be necessary.

Additionally, troubleshooting should involve revisiting the statistical analysis of data. Outliers or anomalies in results might indicate issues with data handling or interpretation. Using appropriate statistical methods and reviewing data for consistency can help identify and address these problems.

In summary, addressing common issues in cytotoxicity testing involves careful attention to sample preparation, reagent quality, equipment maintenance, and data analysis. By systematically troubleshooting these aspects, researchers can enhance the reliability of their cytotoxicity assessments and ensure that their findings are both accurate and reproducible.

9. Future directions in cytotoxicity testing

Future directions in cytotoxicity testing are poised to be shaped by emerging technologies, integration with omics approaches, and advancements in personalized medicine. Innovations in assay technologies are continually enhancing our ability to evaluate cell viability and toxicity with greater precision and efficiency. New methodologies, such as high-content screening and organ-on-a-chip models, offer advanced capabilities for assessing complex cellular responses in more physiologically relevant environments. These technologies enable researchers to simulate more accurately how cells react to various compounds, providing deeper insights into cytotoxic mechanisms and improving the predictive power of assays.

The integration of cytotoxicity assays with omics approaches—such as genomics, proteomics, and metabolomics—holds significant promise for advancing our understanding of cell responses to toxic substances. By combining high-throughput omics data with traditional cytotoxicity assays, researchers can gain a comprehensive view of the molecular changes and pathways affected by toxic compounds. This integration can reveal novel biomarkers for toxicity, uncover new mechanisms of action, and facilitate more accurate risk assessments, ultimately leading to more targeted and effective therapeutic interventions [35].

Personalized medicine stands to benefit greatly from advancements in cytotoxicity testing. By tailoring cytotoxicity assays to individual patient profiles—such as genetic, proteomic, or metabolic characteristics—researchers can develop more personalized therapeutic strategies. This approach allows for the identification of individuals who are most likely to respond to specific treatments or who may be at higher risk of adverse effects, thereby optimizing treatment efficacy and minimizing harm.

However, several challenges and opportunities lie ahead in the field of cytotoxicity testing. One challenge is the need for standardization and validation of new technologies to ensure their reliability and reproducibility. As assays become more sophisticated, integrating them into existing regulatory frameworks and ensuring they meet rigorous standards will be crucial. Additionally, there is a need for interdisciplinary collaboration to fully realize the potential of emerging technologies and omics integration. Opportunities exist to leverage advancements in computational tools and data analytics to enhance the interpretation of complex cytotoxicity data and to drive innovation in assay development.

In summary, the future of cytotoxicity testing is marked by exciting advancements in technology and methodology, promising greater precision and relevance in toxicity assessments. Integrating these innovations with omics data and personalized medicine approaches offers the potential for more effective and individualized therapeutic strategies. Addressing the challenges of standardization and validation while seizing opportunities for interdisciplinary collaboration will be key to advancing the field and improving the impact of cytotoxicity testing on health and medicine [36].

10. Conclusions

In conclusion, this chapter has provided a thorough examination of various cytotoxicity assays, ranging from traditional methods like the MTT assay to modern approaches such as the ATP assay and flow cytometry. We explored the principles, procedures, advantages, limitations, and applications of each assay, highlighting their individual contributions to understanding cell viability and death mechanisms. Additionally, we addressed the interconnectivity between different cell death pathways and discussed how combining assays can offer a more comprehensive assessment of cytotoxicity. This approach not only enhances the accuracy of results but also provides a more nuanced understanding of cellular responses to toxic compounds.

Accurate cytotoxicity assessment is crucial for advancing research and development, particularly in drug discovery, toxicological evaluation, and therapeutic development. By employing a range of assays and integrating new technologies with omics approaches, researchers can obtain a holistic view of how cells respond to various treatments. This comprehensive assessment is vital for identifying potential risks, optimizing therapeutic strategies, and ensuring the safety and efficacy of new compounds.

For researchers, implementing effective cytotoxicity testing strategies involves careful consideration of assay selection based on experimental goals, resources, and cell types. Combining different assays, staying abreast of emerging technologies, and adhering to best practices in assay implementation will significantly enhance the reliability and relevance of cytotoxicity assessments. It is also important to remain adaptable and open to integrating new methodologies and technologies that can provide deeper insights into cell death mechanisms and improve the overall quality of research outcomes.

In summary, a rigorous and multi-faceted approach to cytotoxicity testing is essential for advancing scientific knowledge and ensuring the safety and efficacy of new treatments. By leveraging a diverse array of assays and embracing emerging innovations, researchers can achieve more accurate and meaningful results, ultimately contributing to better health outcomes and more effective therapeutic interventions.

Acknowledgements

The author acknowledges the use of AI tools for the language polishing of the manuscript.

Conflict of interest

The authors declare no conflict of interest.

Author details

Mitali Singhal[1*], Sabita Shaha[2] and Maria Katsikogianni[3]

1 Oxford College of Sciences, Bangalore, India

2 University of Bradford, UK

3 Faculty of Life Sciences, Department of Biomaterials Chemistry, School of Chemistry, University of Bradford, UK

*Address all correspondence to: mitali3005@gmail.com

References

[1] Çelik TA. Introductory Chapter: Cytotoxicity. London, UK: InTechOpen; 2018. DOI: 10.5772/intechopen.77244

[2] Aslantürk ZS. In Vitro Cytotoxicity and Cell Viability Assays: Principles, Advantages, and Disadvantages. London, UK: InTechOpen; 2018. DOI: 10.5772/intechopen.71923

[3] Lewis MA, Patil K, Ettayebi K, Estes MK, Atmar RL, Ramani S. Divergent responses of human intestinal organoid monolayers using commercial in vitro cytotoxicity assays. PLoS One. 2024;**19**(6):e0304526. DOI: 10.1371/journal.pone.0304526

[4] Kroemer G, Galluzzi L, Vandenabeele P, Abrams J, Alnemri E, Baehrecke EH, et al. Classification of cell death: Recommendations of the nomenclature committee on cell death 2009. Cell Death and Differentiation. 2008;**16**(1):3-11. DOI: 10.1038/cdd.2008.150

[5] Goodwin AM. In vitro assays of angiogenesis for assessment of angiogenic and anti-angiogenic agents. Microvascular Research. 2007;**74**(2-3):172-183. DOI: 10.1016/j.mvr.2007.05.006

[6] Jain AK, Singh D, Dubey K, Maurya R, Mittal S, Pandey AK. Models and Methods for In Vitro Toxicity. Elsevier; 2018. pp. 45-65. DOI: 10.1016/b978-0-12-804667-8.00003-1

[7] Ghasemi M, Turnbull T, Sebastian S, Kempson I. The MTT assay: Utility, limitations, pitfalls, and interpretation in bulk and single-cell analysis. International Journal of Molecular Sciences. 2021;**22**(23):12827. DOI: 10.3390/ijms222312827

[8] Marks DC, Belov L, Davey MW, Davey RA, Kidman AD. The MTT cell viability assay for cytotoxicity testing in multidrug-resistant human leukemic cells. Leukemia Research. 1992;**16**(12):1165-1173. DOI: 10.1016/0145-2126(92)90114-m

[9] Bahuguna A, Khan I, Bajpai VK, Kang SC. MTT assay to evaluate the cytotoxic potential of a drug. Bangladesh Journal of Pharmacology. 2017;**12**(2). DOI: 10.3329/bjp.v12i2.30892

[10] Kaja S, Payne AJ, Naumchuk Y, Koulen P. Quantification of lactate dehydrogenase for cell viability testing using cell lines and primary cultured astrocytes. Current Protocols in Toxicology. 2017;**72**(1). DOI: 10.1002/cptx.21

[11] Cox MC, Mendes R, Silva F, Mendes TF, Zelaya-Lazo A, Halwachs K, et al. Application of LDH assay for therapeutic efficacy evaluation of ex vivo tumor models. Scientific Reports. 2021;**11**(1). DOI: 10.1038/s41598-021-97894-0

[12] Kaja S, Payne AJ, Singh T, Ghuman JK, Sieck EG, Koulen P. An optimized lactate dehydrogenase release assay for screening of drug candidates in neuroscience. Journal of Pharmacological and Toxicological Methods. 2015;**73**:1-6. DOI: 10.1016/j.vascn.2015.02.001

[13] Strober W. Trypan blue exclusion test of cell viability. Current Protocols in Immunology. 2015;**111**(1). DOI: 10.1002/0471142735.ima03bs111

[14] Sakowicz-Burkiewicz M, Kocbuch K, Grden M, Maciejewska I, Szutowicz A, Pawelczyk T. High glucose concentration impairs ATP outflow and

immunoglobulin production by human peripheral B lymphocytes: Involvement of P2X7 receptor. Immunobiology. 2013b;**218**(4):591-601. DOI: 10.1016/j.imbio.2012.07.010

[15] McElroy W, Green A. Function of adenosine triphosphate in the activation of luciferin. Archives of Biochemistry and Biophysics. 1956;**64**(2):257-271. DOI: 10.1016/0003-9861(56)90268-5

[16] McKinnon KM. Flow cytometry: An overview. Current Protocols in Immunology. 2018;**120**(1). DOI: 10.1002/cpim.40

[17] Fleisher TA, Oliveira JB. Flow Cytometry. Elsevier; 2019. pp. 1239-1251.e1. DOI: 10.1016/b978-0-7020-6896-6.00092-2

[18] Barteneva NS, Fasler-Kan E, Vorobjev IA. Imaging flow cytometry. Journal of Histochemistry & Cytochemistry. 2012;**60**(10):723-733. DOI: 10.1369/0022155412453052

[19] Leipold MD, Newell EW, Maecker HT. Multiparameter phenotyping of human PBMCs using mass cytometry. Methods in Molecular Biology. 2015:81-95. DOI: 10.1007/978-1-4939-2963-4_7

[20] Mei HE, Leipold MD, Maecker HT. Platinum-conjugated antibodies for application in mass cytometry. Cytometry Part A. 2015;**89**(3):292-300. DOI: 10.1002/cyto.a.22778

[21] Siddiqui S, Livák F. Principles of advanced flow cytometry: A practical guide. Methods in Molecular Biology. 2022:89-114. DOI: 10.1007/978-1-0716-2740-2_5

[22] Jin Z, El-Deiry WS. Overview of cell death signaling pathways. Cancer Biology & Therapy. 2005;**4**(2):147-171. DOI: 10.4161/cbt.4.2.1508

[23] Préaudat M, Ouled-Diaf J, Alpha-Bazin B, Mathis G, Mitsugi T, Aono Y, et al. A homogeneous Caspase-3 activity assay using HTRF® technology. SLAS Discovery. 2002;**7**(3):267-274. DOI: 10.1177/108705710200700310

[24] Nichani K, Li J, Suzuki M, Houston JP. Evaluation of Caspase-3 activity during apoptosis with fluorescence lifetime-based cytometry measurements and phasor analyses. Cytometry Part A. 2020;**97**(12):1265-1275. DOI: 10.1002/cyto.a.24207

[25] Singh R, Letai A, Sarosiek K. Regulation of apoptosis in health and disease: The balancing act of BCL-2 family proteins. Nature Reviews Molecular Cell Biology. 2019;**20**(3):175-193. DOI: 10.1038/s41580-018-0089-8

[26] Mizushima N. Autophagy: Process and function. Genes & Development. 2007;**21**(22):2861-2873. DOI: 10.1101/gad.1599207

[27] Liu S, Yao S, Yang H, Liu S, Wang Y. Autophagy: Regulator of cell death. Cell Death and Disease. 2023;**14**(10). DOI: 10.1038/s41419-023-06154-8

[28] Deretic V. Autophagy in inflammation, infection, and immunometabolism. Immunity. 2021;**54**(3):437-453. DOI: 10.1016/j.immuni.2021.01.018

[29] Levine B, Mizushima N, Virgin HW. Autophagy in immunity and inflammation. Nature. 2011;**469**(7330):323-335. DOI: 10.1038/nature09782

[30] Guiney SJ, Adlard PA, Bush AI, Finkelstein DI, Ayton S. Ferroptosis and cell death mechanisms in Parkinson's disease. Neurochemistry International. 2017;**104**:34-48. DOI: 10.1016/j.neuint.2017.01.004

[31] Vandenabeele P, Vanden Berghe T, Takahashi N. Necroptosis: A Novel Way of Regulated Necrosis with Large Pathophysiological Implications. Elsevier; 2014. pp. 153-161. DOI: 10.1016/b978-0-12-386456-7.01412-x

[32] Stillwell W. Cell Death, Apoptosis. Elsevier; 2016. pp. 539-546. DOI: 10.1016/b978-0-444-63772-7.00024-5

[33] Mattson MP, Culmsee C, Yu ZF. Apoptotic and antiapoptotic mechanisms in stroke. Cell and Tissue Research. 2000;**301**(1):173-187. DOI: 10.1007/s004419900154

[34] Galluzzi L, Kepp O, Krautwald S, Kroemer G, Linkermann A. Molecular mechanisms of regulated necrosis. Seminars in Cell and Developmental Biology. 2014;**35**:24-32. DOI: 10.1016/j.semcdb.2014.02.006

[35] Bhattacharya S, Zhang Q, Carmichael PL, Boekelheide K, Andersen ME. Toxicity testing in the 21st century: Defining new risk assessment approaches based on perturbation of intracellular toxicity pathways. PLoS One. 2011;**6**(6):e20887. DOI: 10.1371/journal.pone.0020887

[36] Krewski D, Andersen ME, Tyshenko MG, Krishnan K, Hartung T, Boekelheide K, et al. Toxicity testing in the 21st century: Progress in the past decade and future perspectives. Archives of Toxicology. 2019;**94**(1):1-58. DOI: 10.1007/s00204-019-02613-4